Cosmetic Make-up and Manicure – The Art and the Science

Ann Eaton, M.C.Dip.H.C. Cert. Ed. and
Florence Openshaw, B.Sc.

PEARSON
Longman

Harlow, England • London • New York • Boston • San Francisco • Toronto
Sydney • Tokyo • Singapore • Hong Kong • Seoul • Taipei • New Delhi
Cape Town • Madrid • Mexico City • Amsterdam • Munich • Paris • Milan

Pearson Education Limited
Edinburgh Gate
Harlow
Essex CM20 2JE
England

and Associated Companies throughout the world

Visit us on the World Wide Web at:
http://www.pearsoned.co.uk

First published 1988

British Library Cataloguing in Publication Data

Eaton. Ann
    Cosmetic make-up and manicure.
    1. Women. Face. Cosmetics. Use. Techniques
    2. Women. Hands. Beauty care
    I. Title   II. Openshaw, Florence
    646.7'26

ISBN 978-0-582-41631-4

22   21   20   19
09   08   07

Set in Linotron 202 Times Roman 9½/11
Printed in Malaysia, GPS

Contents

Part 1 Introduction

Part 2 Cosmetic make-up

Part 3 Manicure

Preface

Cosmetic make-up and manicure are practical arts which require a sound scientific background if they are to be carried out with true understanding. By integrating the art and the relevant science, the authors hope to make the study of these subjects both interesting and meaningful. The book is designed to give students an easily understood introduction to make-up and manicure while preparing for the City and Guilds of London Institute examinations in those subjects and should fill a long-felt need for a suitable text to cover the two topics.

The number of hairdressing salons offering make-up and manicure treatments has increased in recent years, so widening the scope of their services. It is hoped that this book will help many young people to enter this modern leisure industry which offers potentially good prospects for a satisfying career, as well as being a useful source of reference for those already employed in salons.

Acknowledgements

The authors would like to especially thank Nina Eaton, Lecturer at Nelson and Colne College, for both modelling for photographs and for her constructive criticism of the manicure section of the book; Vicky Jarvis, Head of Department of Hairdressing and Beauty Therapy, Northampton College of Further Education, for information and advice; Sidney Kelly of Leebank Proofers, Birmingham, for the supply of diagrams; Sharon Wood for the production of photographs of salon treatments; and Christopher Woodhead of Mercia Beauty Products, Rochdale, for photographs and technical advice. We also wish to express our gratitude to our respective husbands for their support and encouragement and, indeed, for their contribution to the effort involved in producing the manuscript.

In addition, the authors and publishers acknowledge their appreciation to the following for permission to reproduce photographs:

The Boots Company PLC for 'Fantasy make-up' in the colour plate section; Estee Lauder Cosmetics Ltd. for the 'Day make-up' and 'Evening make-up'; in the colour plate section; Caroline Neville Associates (Malvala) for 'Completed manicure' in the colour plate section; Daneglow International, Ilford, Essex for our Fig. 5.7; Institute of Dermatology for our Figs. 6.2, 6.3, 6.4, 6.5, 6.6, 6.7, 17.15 and 17.16, Mercia Beauty Products, Rochdale for our Figs. 1.1, 1.2 and 14.2.

Part 1
Introduction

Chapter 1

The salon

Cosmetic make-up and manicure treatments are frequently offered as additional services in hairdressing salons. The salon itself should have a pleasant relaxing atmosphere rather than being clinical or austere. Clients appreciate a certain amount of luxury and a well thought-out colour scheme with toning furnishings, gowns and towels will help to provide an attractive environment. Safety in the salon is important, too, so that equipment should be of a high standard, be kept in good repair and carefully sited in order to avoid accidents. The salon should be well lit, have an efficient system of ventilation and be comfortably maintained at a temperature between 21–24 °C. Strict attention must be paid to salon hygiene.

Basic equipment

A certain amount of basic equipment is required if services are to be carried out in conditions of comfort for both clients and staff. In addition to suitable furniture, many smaller items such as towels, bowls, tissues and cotton wool are required along with cosmetic and manicure preparations and tools.

For cosmetic make-up, a chair which will tilt and which has some neck support or, alternatively, a couch is advisable, since the client's head and shoulders should be well supported during treatment. A tray or trolley to hold cosmetic preparations and small items of equipment is also required, and a suitable mirror should be readily available.

For manicure treatment the basic equipment consists of a table or preferably a trolley to hold manicure preparations and tools. Two chairs of suitable height for the manicurist and client are also required. The manicurist must be able to work comfortably without having to bend unduly, so avoiding possible fatigue in the muscles of the back.

Small tools and items of equipment for make-up and manicure are illustrated and listed in Fig. 1.1 and Fig. 1.2. Make-up brushes are shown in Fig. 1.4 and in Fig. 14.2.

In addition, both cosmeticians and manicurists require access to a hot and cold water supply, facilities for the sterilisation of tools and storage space for small items of equipment and towels.

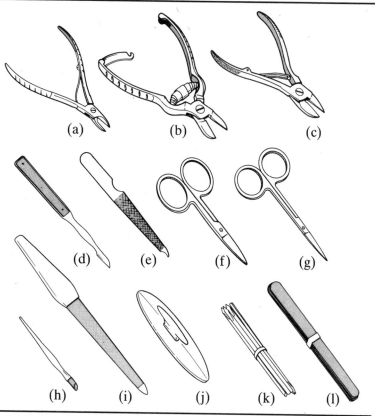

Fig. 1.1 Tools used in manicure

(a) Cuticle pliers, (b) Barrel spring nail pliers, (c) Nail pliers, (d) Cuticle knife, (e) Nail File, (f) Nail scissors, (g) Cuticle scissors, (h) Rubber-ended hoof stick, (i) Sapphire nail file, (j) Nail buffer, (k) Manicure sticks, (l) Emery boards

Stock control

The purpose of efficient stock control is to ensure that:
1. Items of equipment and materials are available as required.
2. Materials are not wasted by misuse, unsuitable storage or by being kept beyond their normal shelf-life.
3. Regular replacement of equipment and stock is carried out to maintain the highest possible standards within the salon.

The stock of a salon may be classified as:
1. **Durables** which include large equipment, e.g. couches, trolleys, sterilising cabinets etc., requiring replacement very infrequently. These should be chosen with care after study of the types of equipment available, possibly from catalogues or at an exhibition or a wholesale

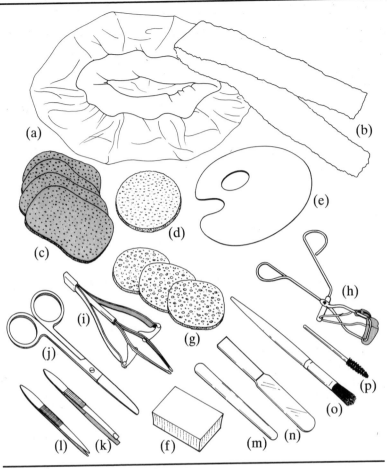

Fig. 1.2 Tools and equipment for make-up

(a) Headband with net crown, (b) Headband with velcro fixing, (c) Mousseline lamellae sponges, (d) Mask-removing sponges, (e) Make-up palette, (f) Make-up wedges, (g) Sponges, (h) Eyelash curler, (i) Automatic tweezers, (j) Nurses scissors, (k) Tweezers, (l) Tweezers pointed, (m) Lip spatula, (n) Plexiglass spatula, (o) Masking brush, (p) Mascara spiral brush

warehouse. The equipment should be suitable for its purpose and capable of withstanding years of continuous use.

2. **Semi-consumables** including smaller items such as towels, nippers, scissors, brushes and bowls which may require periodic renewal. These should be of good quality, and stock should include spare items ready to be brought into use when required.

3. **Consumables** such as cosmetics, manicure products, emery boards, orange sticks, tissues and cotton wool, which require very frequent renewal. Consumables should be bought in bulk since this is the

cheapest method, but too large a stock ties up capital and this should be avoided. Liquids purchased in bulk in large containers are best decanted into smaller vessels for everyday use to avoid waste. To prevent damage to labels, liquids should be poured from bottles on the side away from the label. For cosmetics and manicure products it is advisable to concentrate on more popular lines and colours, always taking into account the needs of regular clients. The items in stock should be kept fairly constant and new products not introduced too frequently. This helps both staff and clients. New products should be purchased in small quantities and tried out first, possibly on staff, before being permanently on the stock list. Gimmicky new products recommended by high-pressure salesmen are best avoided.

4. **Stock for resale to clients**. Care must be taken to avoid excessive stocks which could become unsaleable. This stock should be well displayed in order to catch the client's eye.

The method of stock keeping depends on the size of the salon, but a separate lockable stockroom should be available with one person responsible for stock records and dispensing. A cool, dark room is preferable as heat tends to cause deterioration of products and sunlight may cause coloured goods such as nail enamels to fade. Shelves should be labelled to facilitate the finding of items. Heavy items should be kept at a reasonable height so as to be easily accessible and items used frequently should be placed at eye level.

A stock book should be kept and brought up to date daily to record incoming stock, items used, sales made and stock in hand. This enables re-ordering to be carried out efficiently. In large organisations this may be controlled by computer. Copies should be kept of official orders and goods carefully checked on delivery. The advice note should be retained. Goods not up to standard or not as ordered should be returned to the supplier using a goods returned note and not paid for unless changed. Invoices or statements of account should be kept for checking by the accountant. Advantage should be taken of any discounts offered by suppliers.

When new stock is delivered, the older stock should be moved to the front of the shelf and the newly acquired stock placed at the back, or new stock could be date stamped on arrival and used in rotation. The shelf-life of the product is important, so stocktaking should be carried out at six-monthly intervals, the stock room thoroughly cleaned, and old stock discarded and written out of the stock book. The stockroom floor should be free from clutter and if there is any spillage it should be cleaned away immediately to prevent accidents.

Salon hygiene

Attention to salon hygiene is essential to protect both the operative and the client from infection by micro-organisms such as bacteria, viruses and fungi. There are two methods by which infection may be transferred from one person to another:

1. **By direct contact** with an infected person either by touching an infected area of a person's skin or by inhaling air-borne droplets ejected from the nose or mouth when an infected person is speaking, coughing or sneezing.
2. **By indirect contact** with an infected article. This is a less obvious method of infection and is a great danger in salons unless a high standard of hygiene is maintained. It involves cross-infection which is the passing of infection from a person to an object, e.g. a towel or a jar of cosmetic cream, and subsequent transfer of the infection to a second person. The two people involved may never actually meet and could have entered the salon on completely different occasions.

To avoid infection by direct contact:

1. The operative's hands must be washed immediately before attention to a client so that infection is not passed directly to the client's skin.
2. The operative's hands must be washed again immediately on completion of treatment to remove any infection passed from the client's skin to the hands.
3. The salon operative must never touch a client's skin if it is considered that infection may be present, e.g. warts, cold sores, boils and impetigo sores should not be touched. If necessary the client should be advised to consult a doctor.
4. Staff with heavy colds or other infections should stay away from the salon to avoid passing on infection. Air-borne infection may be minimised by good ventilation.

To avoid infection by indirect contact:

1. The salon operative's hands should be washed before removing tools from an ultra-violet cabinet and setting out equipment for use on a client. This is particularly important after a visit to the toilet or after blowing the nose. Sterilised tools should be held by the handle only and immediately placed either on a clean tissue or in an antiseptic solution.
2. Clean towels, gowns, headbands, tissues and cotton wool should be used for each client and all tools sterilised before use. Couches and chairs used for make-up treatments should be covered with clean towels for each client, especially where a head rest is being utilised. Clean cotton wool should be stored in a closed container.
3. During treatment, sterilised spatulas should be used to remove cream from jars and the cream placed on the back of the operator's non-working hand prior to application on the client. The cap must be replaced on the jar immediately after use to prevent the entry of air-borne dust and germs. This ensures that the cream remaining in

the jar is germ-free and so prevents the possibility of cross-infection. Similar care is necessary to avoid cross-infection when using cake make-up, lipsticks and other cosmetic materials which are to be used on several clients. The required amount of make-up must be removed by spatula on to a sterile palette, and applied to the client with a sterilised brush. Any tool accidentally dropped on to the floor must be re-sterilised before use.

4. When treatment is completed, disposables such as orange sticks and emery boards should be broken so that they cannot be re-used, and then destroyed along with used cotton wool and tissues. Tools such as brushes, manicure implements and tweezers must be cleaned and sterilised before use on the next client. Lip pencils, eyebrow pencils and eyeliners should be re-sharpened to provide a new surface for the next application and kept in an ultra-violet cabinet until required. Small tools not being re-used immediately should be stored in a clean container and preferably covered.

5. The salon itself must be cleaned regularly to remove dust and dirt which may harbour germs. Where possible, surfaces should be disinfected. Salon surfaces are best made from materials which are easily kept clean, are free from crevices and are impervious to water and chemicals. Rubbish bins must be kept covered and the contents preferably burned at the end of the day.

AIDS (Acquired Immune Deficiency Syndrome)

The rapid spread of AIDS has focused attention on hygiene in salons. AIDS is a disease caused by a virus known as HIV (Human Immunodeficiency Virus). This virus attacks those cells in the blood which normally form part of the defence system of the body by producing antibodies to fight infection. The AIDS patient may thus eventually die from any infection which, due to lack of suitable antibodies, the body is unable to fight and overcome.

AIDS may either be transmitted by direct contact during sexual intercourse or by indirect contact through injection of the virus into the blood stream by use of an infected needle. The latter method is usually confined to drug addicts who share unsterilised needles. It could, however, be passed on in a salon during ear-piercing if this were carried out using a previously infected and unsterilised needle. Modern methods of ear-piercing using a gun are safe if correctly used, since pre-sterilised rings are supplied by the manufacturer and only used once.

Although the disease is not thought to be transmitted through cuts, it is wise to allay the client's fears by the careful use of manicure tools and obvious attention to their sterilisation. If a client is accidentally cut, apply antiseptic immediately. Wash any blood from the tool involved, wipe it over with surgical spirit and re-sterilise it immediately. Similarly it is advisable that the manicurist should, as far as possible, prevent the client's blood from coming into contact with her own hands.

The sterilisation of tools

Sterilisation means the complete destruction of living organisms on an object and is rarely achieved in a salon without the use of an autoclave. The terms 'sterilising' and 'sterilising cabinets' are, however, in common use though 'disinfecting' or 'sanitising', which imply a reduction of health hazards without complete sterilisation, may be more accurate.

Micro-organisms (bacteria, viruses and fungi) may be destroyed by heat, chemical disinfectants and ultra-violet radiation. It must be emphasised that all tools should be cleaned to remove grease before disinfection is attempted.

Disinfection by heat

Heat kills micro-organisms by coagulating the protein of which they are composed (rather like the coagulation of egg white in a boiled egg). This usually takes place at about 70 °C, but higher temperatures are required to kill bacterial spores which develop tough coats to help them survive adverse conditions.

1. *Dry heat*. Burning destroys all micro-organisms and is the best way of dealing with salon waste. A naked flame may be used to sterilise small metal tools such as tweezers, but tends to blunt sharp metal edges. Hot air ovens will sterilise objects left at 150 °C for one hour, but the high temperature makes it unsuitable for salon use.

2. *Moist heat*. Boiling in water at 100 °C for 15 minutes is suitable for the disinfection of towels and other cotton goods. Boiling under increased pressure by use of an autoclave, which is similar in action to a pressure cooker, is an effective method of sterilisation, and is used in hospitals and in some beauty salons (see Fig. 1.3).

If water vapour is not allowed to escape from a container in which water is being heated, pressure on the surface of the water is increased. This makes it more difficult for molecules to leave the surface of the water until they are given more energy by raising the

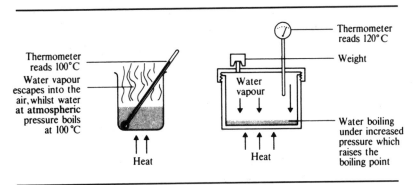

Fig. 1.3 Increasing the pressure raises the boiling point

temperature. Thus increasing the pressure raises the boiling point of water. At normal atmospheric pressure water boils at 100 °C, but on doubling the pressure the boiling point rises to about 120 °C. Autoclaving is suitable for glass and rubber objects.

Chemical disinfectants

A *disinfectant* is a substance which will kill germs when used long enough and strong enough. A weak solution of a disinfectant may in some cases be used as an *antiseptic*, a substance which prevents the multiplication of germs but does not necessarily kill them, and which can be used on the skin to prevent wounds becoming septic. Many disinfectants are unsuitable for use on the skin. Those used in salons include formaldehyde gas, cetrimide and sodium hypochlorite. Antiseptics include hydrogen peroxide (5 vols.), cetrimide and chloroxylenol (Dettol).

Formaldehyde gas is an effective disinfectant commonly used in salons. Its fumes are irritant to the nose and eyes so a special cabinet is required for its use. The manufacturer's instructions regarding use should always be followed. The gas is formed inside the cabinet by heating 5 per cent formalin (methanal) solution using an electrical heater in the base of the cabinet. Brushes, bowls and cosmetic pencils may be sterilised by this method, but must be free from grease and left in the cabinet for at least 20 minutes. Formaldehyde attacks metals and could spoil the cutting edge of metal tools. For this reason, ultra-violet cabinets are more practical for make-up and manicure purposes.

Liquid chemical disinfectants used in salons include:

(a) Quaternary ammonium compounds (Quats) which are among the most effective of modern disinfectants. The one most often used in salons is cetrimide which, as a 1–2 per cent solution, is suitable as a bath for tools. Cetrimide is cationic, so carries a positive electrical charge, and its effectiveness is destroyed by contact with soap or anionic soapless detergents which have a negative charge.

(b) Alcohol (surgical spirit) may be used to clean eyebrow tweezers and other small metal tools before placing them in an ultra-violet cabinet. It is also useful to clean the skin before carrying out predisposition or hypersensitivity tests for eyelash dyes.

(c) Sodium hypochlorite (Milton) is often used by cosmeticians as a sterilising fluid in which to place spatulas after use.

Ultra-violet radiation

Cabinets using ultra-violet radiation (see Fig. 1.4) are exceedingly popular in salons. The ultra-violet rays are produced by a mercury vapour lamp sited at the top of the cabinet. Radiation travels in straight lines so that objects must be frequently turned so that all surfaces obtain the benefit of the rays. However, most professional UV Cabinets have reflective internal surfaces to give some UV treatment to under surfaces

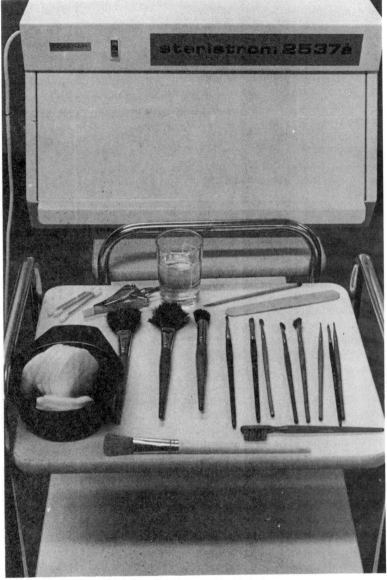

Fig. 1.4 Ultra-violet cabinet. (Courtesy of Coast Air, Sudbury)

too. Objects should also be grease-free as the rays are absorbed by grease. Thus these cabinets are best used for storing equipment which has been previously sterilised by other means. Ultra-violet rays are damaging to the eyes and the lamp switches off automatically as the door opens. The cabinets are suitable for all types of equipment which should be exposed to the rays for at least 20 minutes.

The salon water supply

An adequate supply of both hot and cold water is required in a salon. In addition to that required for treatment purposes such as mixing clay-based face masks or soaking the hands during manicure, water is required for the regular washing of the salon operative's hands, the cleansing of the salon itself and for washing towels, gowns etc.

Cold water enters the salon by an underground mains service pipe bringing water originating as rainwater and usually collected in reservoirs or lakes. This water must be heated in the salon as required, by an electrical immersion heater, instantaneous water heaters or boilers.

While the mains supply has been treated to make it safe for drinking and washing purposes, it is not chemically pure water and may contain various substances which were dissolved in it on its passage through the ground before collection in the reservoir. In some areas water contains sufficient dissolved calcium and magnesium salts to make it 'hard'. When soap is used with hard water an insoluble scum is formed before a lather is obtained. Soft water contains few dissolved salts and will form an immediate lather with soap. In hard water areas the whole of the salon supply may be softened by passing the incoming water through an ion-exchange water softener. In this case the calcium and magnesium salts are replaced by sodium salts which do not react with soap, so that the water is soft.

Hard water is considered to be drying to the skin, and for various salon treatments purified water is preferred, for example in toning facial skin after cleansing and in the preparation of clay-based face masks. Purified water may be purchased for this purpose. Purification is usually carried out by the process of de-ionisation in which water is passed through two separate columns of ion-exchange resins which remove all dissolved salts. Pure water may also be obtained by distillation. Water is boiled to form steam so leaving impurities behind. The steam is then cooled and pure water is collected.

Questions

1. Discuss the importance of clean hands for salon operatives. At what stages and for what reasons should the hands be washed during preparation of the salon and treatment of clients?
2. Explain the difference between each of the following:
   (a) sterilisation and sanitisation;
   (b) a disinfectant and an antiseptic;
   (c) hard and soft water;

(d) distilled and de-ionised water.
3. What is meant by cross-infection? What steps may be taken to avoid cross-infection in a salon?
4. How would you treat the following items after use:
   (a) cuticle nippers;   (b) orange sticks;   (c) towels;   (d) lip pencils?
5. Describe how a stockroom could best be arranged to provide easy access to stores.

Chapter 2

Client relationship

A good relationship between salon operatives and their clients is of prime importance for a successful business. To attain this relationship the operative must cultivate a professional attitude in communicating with the client and impress the client by having a well-groomed appearance and a consistently pleasant manner. Every care should be taken to ensure that the client is comfortable and relaxed while in the salon.

Client reception

The client's first impression of a salon and its staff is of the utmost importance for a first impression is a lasting one. A clean and tidy reception area and a smart businesslike receptionist with a pleasant and welcoming manner will put the client at ease. Each client requires a personal service. She must always be addressed by name and her needs anticipated. The salon staff should always show their clients every consideration. The aim should be to provide an efficient yet enjoyable service in a relaxed and friendly atmosphere. If the client has to wait for treatment, her coat should be taken and a seat and magazine offered. Waiting time, however, should be as short as possible and an accurate system of appointments will ensure a steady flow of clients which will give staff time to work at a reasonable speed without undue pressure and allow time for conversation with the client. The sequence of the day's programme for the salon should be worked out carefully and record cards, equipment and stock made ready before the client arrives for treatment. The use of record cards enables a second person to continue treatment in the absence of the usual operator and makes the client feel more valued.

Telephone bookings must be dealt with efficiently but pleasantly. The exact type of treatment required should be noted along with the appointment time and name of client. If advice is asked, the receptionist should be able to respond with details of treatments, cost of service and the time required for treatment.

Client comfort

Whether carrying out a make-up or a manicure, it is essential that the client remains comfortable and relaxed throughout the treatment. *To ensure client comfort during make-up:*

1. The cosmetician should:
   (a) avoid wearing rings or bracelets since these may scratch the client or cause pain and other discomfort during treatment;
   (b) maintain the highest possible standard of personal hygiene to avoid giving offence to the client;
   (c) keep her own nails short;
   (d) ensure that her hands are warm before touching the client's skin;
   (e) ensure that tools and equipment are scrupulously clean, since lack of hygiene may lead to an apprehensive client.
2. The salon itself should be:
   (a) kept warm, well ventilated and quiet;
   (b) adequately lit without subjecting the client to the glare of badly placed lights.
3. The client should:
   (a) always be positioned comfortably whether fully reclining or seated upright;
   (b) have adequate protection for both her clothing and hair.
4. During treatment:
   (a) the client's skin must always be treated gently, particularly round the eyes;
   (b) sufficient cleansing cream should be used to ensure a comfortable massage without dragging the skin;
   (c) the client should be warned if the product to be used will feel either cold or hot; for example, astringent lotions and some face packs may feel cold, while paraffin wax masks and oil masks will feel warm.
   (d) care should be taken to avoid startling the client during treatments when her eyes are closed or eyepads are being worn; the client must be warned whenever the cosmetician intends to touch her skin, remove the pads or proceed with any further treatment.

To ensure client comfort during manicure:
1. The manicurist should:
   (a) avoid wearing jewellery on the wrists and hands, since this may scratch the client or cause discomfort during hand massage;
   (b) maintain a high standard of personal hygiene to avoid causing offence to the client;
   (c) ensure that treatments are carried out in hygienic surroundings.
2. The salon itself should be warm and well ventilated.
3. The client should:
   (a) be seated comfortably;
   (b) have her cuffs or sleeves turned back and kept away from manicure products which may stain the clothing;
   (c) be asked to remove jewellery from her hands (this must be kept safely but within the client's view throughout the treatment).
4. During treatment:
   (a) manicure products and tools should be suitably placed so that the manicurist does not constantly reach over in front of the client;

(b) the client's hands and arms must be well supported, particularly during the massage procedure;

(c) sufficient cream should be used during the massage to avoid discomfort to the client;

(d) water used for soaking the client's fingers must be warm;

(e) oils and paraffin wax used during remedial treatments must not be too hot;

(f) great care should be taken when using cuticle cutting tools so that no damage occurs to the cuticle, surrounding skin or to the nail plate.

Social skills

A trained and experienced member of the salon staff will show skill in handling clients so that the client is given confidence, feels relaxed and ready to enjoy the treatment. While offering advice about the most suitable and beneficial treatment, the salon operative must always be prepared to follow the client's wishes and personal preferences. A calm but efficient manner will enable problems to be dealt with if they arise. The client may require tactful advice regarding contra-indications to treatment or the necessity of consulting a doctor about a particular condition.

Conversation with the client may be limited during some make-up treatment but in general the amount depends on the client herself and the salon operative should follow her lead. Some clients prefer the stimulation of constant conversation while others prefer a quieter and more relaxed visit. Controversial subjects such as religion and politics must always be avoided. Personal comments concerning clients should not be made and sexual matters not discussed. It is important to be a good listener without feeling obliged to give advice about personal problems. At all times the confidence of the client must be respected and information obtained from a client should not be repeated. Any information given by the client regarding her own health should be mentally noted since it may be useful to know in an emergency that a particular client has, for example, a heart condition or is diabetic or asthmatic.

Courtesy should be extended to the client from the moment of entering the salon, throughout the treatment period, to the moment of leaving. A satisfied client is the best possible advertisement for a salon as the client's recommendation will be passed on to others.

Appearance and deportment

The personal appearance of the salon operative and the way she walks, stands and sits are important in creating a good professional image. A neat, tidy and well-groomed operative, appropriately but immaculately dressed in a clean overall kept in good repair, gives an immediate impression of efficiency. The hair should be kept short and tidy and not allowed to fall over the client or the equipment. Similarly, dangling jewellery should be avoided. The hands are particularly important since they are constantly in the client's view during treatment. They should be well manicured with finger nails of a practical length. The skin of the hands should be kept soft and supple by the regular use of hand cream at night. Make-up should not be too heavy and the excessive use of perfume should be avoided.

Bad posture in a salon operative gives clients an impression of an unenthusiastic worker as well as possibly leading to ill-health or fatigue. Clothes also do not look their best and may hang unevenly since they are made to fit a well-balanced figure.

Cosmeticians often have to stand while carrying out treatments and it is important that the client is at the correct height so that too much bending is avoided. Posture during standing is correct if a straight line can be drawn from the mastoid process of the temporal bone just behind the ear, through the tip of the shoulder and the mid-line of the hips to the front of the knee and the front of the ankle (see Fig. 2.1). Fatigue may be caused if one part of the body is out of line with the part immediately below it since this puts strain on the ligaments which bind the bones together.

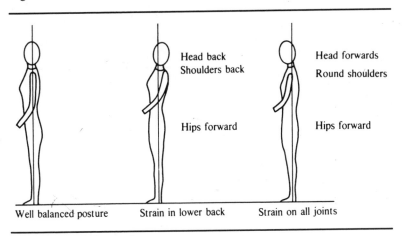

Well balanced posture   Strain in lower back   Strain on all joints

Fig. 2.1 Posture during standing

The shoulders should be level and point straight out at the sides. If the shoulders are held too far back the natural curve of the back is flattened and this causes tension in the lower back. Holding the shoulders forwards compresses the chest and restricts the circulation and respiration, also causing the upper part of the back to become rounded. The head should be held straight up. If the chin drops, the line of vision is changed. If the chin is pushed outwards, the head tilts back causing strain in the neck and shoulder muscles. Holding the head on one side causes tension in the neck muscles, as well as affecting vision since the eyes are on different levels.

To habitually stand with the weight on one foot is bad practice as this strains the ligaments of the spine (see Fig. 2.2). In standing, the feet should be a little distance apart so that the legs are vertical or straight down from the hips. The toes should point straight forwards in both standing and walking, so that the body weight falls on the flat outer edges of the foot and not on the arches.

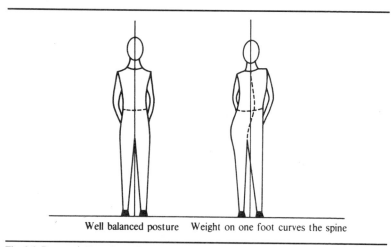

Well balanced posture   Weight on one foot curves the spine

Fig. 2.2 Posture (effect of standing with the weight on one foot)

Foot discomfort may affect the ability to stand and walk correctly. A chiropodist should be consulted for treatment of painful conditions such as ingrowing toe nails, corns, bunions and plantar warts (verrucae). Well-fitting shoes are also essential. They should grip at the heels and over the instep. The arches of the feet should be supported and there should be room for the toes to move easily inside the shoes. Very high heels tend to throw the body forwards and may lead to bad posture; a low or medium heel is usually more comfortable.

Manicurists, who usually sit while carrying out treatments, should adopt an elegant position by sitting well back in the chair with the weight of the body supported by the pelvis rather than the bottom of the spine. The thighs should be supported by the chair itself, but some of their weight should also be borne by the feet or there will be pressure on the blood vessels and nerves at the backs of the thighs. There should be a right-angle at the knee joint and the feet should be together and flat on the floor. To avoid strain, the back should be kept straight while working (see Fig. 2.3).

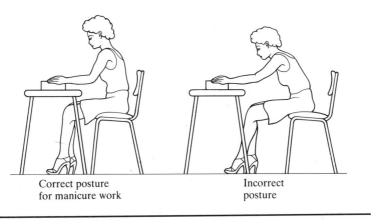

Correct posture
for manicure work

Incorrect
posture

Fig. 2.3 Posture while sitting

Personal hygiene

Attention to personal hygiene is important if the salon operative is not to cause offence to clients by perspiration and breath odours. There are two sources of perspiration:

1. *Eccrine or sudoriferous glands* are present in most parts of the skin and secrete perspiration consisting of 98 per cent water and about 2 per cent sodium chloride (common salt) with traces of waste products such as urea and lactic acid.
2. *Apocrine sweat glands* are located mostly in the armpits and pubic area and secrete perspiration with a more fatty content than eccrine sweat. This type of perspiration is readily attacked by bacteria which break down the sweat into substances with an unpleasant odour.

A daily bath or shower is necessary to remove both types of sweat as well as dead skin, dirt, bacteria and excess sebum. Underclothing which absorbs perspiration should also be changed daily.

Underarm sweating may be reduced by the use of antiperspirant lotions which are packaged as 'roll-on' lotions, squeeze sprays and aerosols. The lotions contain astringents such as aluminium chlorhydrate, and deodorants in the form of antiseptics such as cetrimide or hexachlorophene which prevent the multiplication of the bacteria causing odour by the breakdown of sweat. Talcum powder may also be used as a good absorbent of sweat for both the underarm and for excessive foot perspiration.

Unpleasant breath (halitosis) may be caused by digestive problems or by decay of food particles lodged in pockets in the gums or in decaying teeth. Offence to clients can also be caused by mouth odours from smoking and after eating strong smelling foods such as oranges, curry and garlic. Mouth hygiene involves frequent cleansing of the teeth, regular visits to the dentist and, if necessary, the use of antiseptic mouth washes.

Questions

1. Why is the personal appearance of salon operatives important?
2. What are the characteristics of a good receptionist?
3. In what ways may a salon operative cause offence to a client by neglect of personal hygiene? What steps can the operative take to ensure day-long personal freshness?
4. What considerations govern the conversation between a salon operative and a client?
5. What preparations should be made in a salon before the arrival of the client to ensure that her visit will be comfortable and relaxed?

Part 2
Cosmetic make-up

Chapter 3

Bones and muscles of the head

The shape of the face is an important consideration in deciding the type of make-up required for a client. Face shape is determined by the formation of the facial bones of the skull and the depth of the soft tissue composed of muscle and subcutaneous fat, which lies between the bone and the skin. The appearance of the face itself changes with the years. The gradual development of expression lines in facial skin, caused by the repeated contraction of facial muscles, is one of the first signs of an ageing skin.

The bones of the skull

The skull consists of twenty-two bones and may be considered in two parts, the *cranium* and the *face*. The cranium, a protective box holding the brain, is made up of eight bones. The face is composed of fourteen bones. The only movable bone in the skull is the lower jaw or mandible which is hinged to allow chewing and talking to take place. All the other bones are held rigidly together by saw-edged joints called *sutures*.

The bones of the cranium

The bones forming the cranium are shown in Fig. 3.1 and Fig. 3.2 and they are as follows:
1. **The frontal bone** forms the forehead and the front part of the top of the cranium. It contains two large air cavities or sinuses connected to the nasal cavities by small openings, making the bones lighter and giving resonance to the voice. The sinus linings sometimes become infected following a cold.
2. **A pair of parietal bones** join down the mid-line of the top of the cranium forming the top and part of the sides of the cranium.
3. **The occipital bone** forms the back and part of the base of the cranium. It contains a large opening, the foramen magnum, through which passes the spinal cord.
4. **A pair of temporal bones** form the lower part of the sides of the cranium and contain cavities for the ear passages. A portion of each temporal bone juts out to join the corresponding cheek bone, forming

the zygomatic arches which can be felt on each side of the face in front of the lower part of the ear.

5. **The sphenoid bone** occupies most of the base of the cranium. It is shaped like a bat with its extended wing tips forming part of each side of the cranium, between the temporal and frontal bones.

6. **The ethmoid bone** is a small irregularly shaped bone which forms part of the base of the cranium, the roof of the nose and the inner wall of the *orbits* (eye sockets). This bone is not shown in the diagrams.

The bones of the face (see Fig. 3.1 and Fig. 3.2)

Although there are fourteen bones in the face, only seven of them affect the shape of the face. These are as follows:

1. **A pair of small nasal bones** form the bridge of the nose. The rest of the nose contains cartilage which is much softer and more flexible than bone. The cartilage determines the shape of the lower part of the nose.

2. **A pair of zygomatic bones** (malar) form the cheek bones. The zygomatic arches join the cheek bones to the temporal bones, on each side of the face. The position of the zygomatic bones can easily be found by following the zygomatic arches down on to the face. The cheek bones will be felt protruding above the upper jaw bones.

3. **Two superior maxillary bones or maxillae** form the upper jaw, part of the roof of the mouth, and also hold the upper teeth.

4. **The inferior maxillary bone or mandible** forms the lower jaw and holds the lower teeth. It connects with the temporal bone, making a movable joint to enable chewing and talking to take place.

The other seven facial bones (two lachrymal bones in the orbits, two turbinate bones behind the nose, two palatine bones in the roof of the mouth and the vomer which forms part of the septum between the nostrils) have no influence on the shape of the face and are not included in the diagrams.

The muscles of the head and neck

The bones of the face are covered with layers of muscle or flesh which, together with the skin and its underlying layer of subcutaneous fat, give roundness to the contours of the face. Each muscle consists of a bundle of contractile fibres enclosed in a sheath of fibrous tissue, which narrows towards the ends of the muscles to form the *tendon* which attaches the muscle to bone or skin. Muscles work by contracting in length; they can pull but never push. Contraction of muscle fibres results in the movement of a bone or skin. For example, the lower jaw is raised by contraction of the muscles of mastication, and wrinkling of the skin as in frowning is caused by the contraction of the supercilii muscles in the forehead.

The contraction of muscles depends on nerve impulses carried from

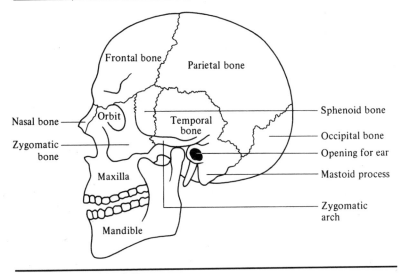

Fig. 3.1 Side view of the skull

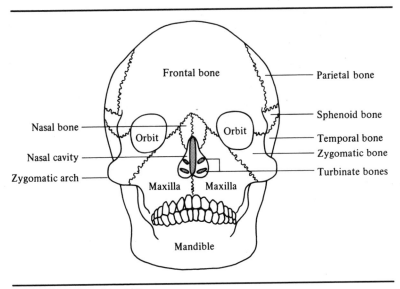

Fig. 3.2 Front view of the skull

the brain along motor nerves. Supplies of glucose and oxygen are also necessary to produce energy for the contraction and these are brought to the muscle by the arterial blood system. Thus muscles always need an adequate blood and nerve supply (see Fig. 3.3).

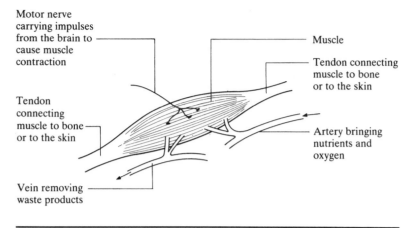

Motor nerve carrying impulses from the brain to cause muscle contraction

Tendon connecting muscle to bone or to the skin

Vein removing waste products

Muscle

Tendon connecting muscle to bone or to the skin

Artery bringing nutrients and oxygen

Fig. 3.3 Blood and nerve supply to a muscle

The chief muscles of the head and neck (see Fig. 3.4 and Fig. 3.5) fall into three groups:
1. The muscles of mastication.
2. The muscles which move the head.
3. The muscles of facial expression.

The muscles of mastication

The *masseter* and the *temporalis* muscles are the chief muscles of mastication. The masseters extend from the zygomatic arch to the angle of the lower jaw on each side of the face. Contraction of the muscles raises the lower jaw and clenches the teeth. The temporalis muscles are fan shaped and extend from the temporal bones to the lower jaw on each side of the face. Contraction of the temporalis muscles raises the jaw, draws it backwards if protruding, and allows the jaw to move from side to side in grinding movements.

The muscles which move the head

The *sternomastoid* and *trapezius* muscles are responsible for head movements. The sternomastoid muscles extend from the breast bone or sternum to the mastoid process which is part of the temporal bone and is situated just behind the ears. The muscles thus pass one on each side of the neck. When both muscles contract together, the head moves down as in nodding. When used singly the head is turned to the side opposite to the contracting muscle.

The trapezius muscles are broad flat muscles extending from the occipital bone at the back of the skull to the shoulder blades, and thus cover

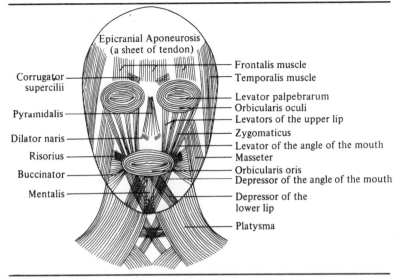

Fig. 3.4 Muscles of the head and neck (front view)

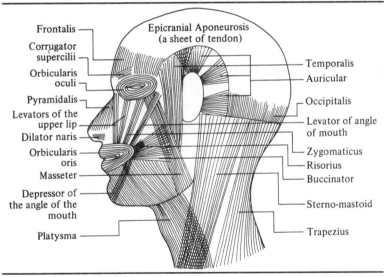

Fig. 3.5 Muscles of the head and neck (side view)

the back of the neck. The two muscles used together draw the head backwards. Contraction of one of the muscles only draws the head to the side of the contracting muscle. These muscles may also be used to raise the shoulders.

The muscles of facial expression

The main muscles of facial expression are listed in Table 3.1.

Table 3.1 The muscles of facial expression

Group	Name of muscle	Position	Action
Muscles of lips and cheeks	Orbicularis oris	Circular muscle round the mouth	Closes the mouth. Used in talking and whistling
	Risorius	Radiates from the corner of the mouth	Causes smiling
	Buccinator	Inside cheeks	Keeps food between the teeth during mastication Puffs out the cheeks as in blowing
	Levator of upper lip	Radiates from upper lip	Raises upper lip
	Zygomaticus	Radiates from upper lip	Raises upper lip
	Levator of angle of mouth	Radiates from upper lip	Raises corners of the mouth
	Depressor of the lower lip	Radiates from lower lip	Draws down the lower lip
	Depressor of the angle of mouth	Radiates from lower lip	Draws down corner of the mouth
	Mentalis	Radiates from lower lip	Turns lower lip outwards
Muscles of forehead	Frontalis	Attached to epicranial aponeurosis	Wrinkles forehead horizontally and moves the scalp
	Corrugator supercilii	Small muscles under eyebrows	Vertical wrinkles in forehead (frowning)
Muscles of eye area	Orbicularis oculi	Circular muscle round eye	Closes eyelids
	Levator palpebrae	In upper eyelids	Opens upper eyelids
Muscles of ears	Auricular muscles	Group of muscles behind the ears	Moves ears slightly (in some people)
Muscles of nose	Pyramidalis	On front of nose	Wrinkles nose
	Dilator naris	Side of nostrils	Dilates nostrils
Muscles of neck	Platysma	Sheet of muscle under skin of neck	Used in sudden fear or looking fierce

Many muscles concerned with facial expression are attached at both ends to the skin of the face rather than to bones of the skull. In some cases the pull of the muscle on the skin may cause a depression or a dimple. When the facial muscles contract, they wrinkle the skin and throw it into folds since the muscles can contract but the skin cannot (see Fig. 3.6). These wrinkles and folds give rise to a wide variety of facial expressions.

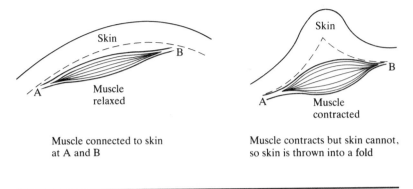

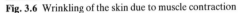

| Muscle connected to skin at A and B | Muscle contracts but skin cannot, so skin is thrown into a fold |

Fig. 3.6 Wrinkling of the skin due to muscle contraction

In youth, the folds disappear on relaxation of the muscles. Later in life, due to repeated contraction of the same muscles and some loss of the skin's elasticity, the skin is unable to return to its original state when the muscles relax and the expression lines become permanent. The appearance of these lines is the first indication of the ageing of the skin. The main expression lines are listed in Table 3.2 along with the muscles responsible for the various lines. These are also shown diagrammatically in Fig. 3.7.

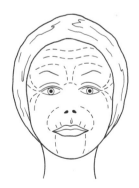

Fig. 3.7 Expression lines

Table 3.2 Expression lines

Expression line	Cause	Muscle involved
Crow's feet (laughter lines) at corners of the eyes	Screwing up the eyes when laughing or in bright sunlight or when smoking	Orbicularis oculi
Horizontal lines on forehead	Raising eyebrows in look of surprise or astonishment	Frontalis
Vertical lines in centre forehead	Frowning	Corrugator supercilii
Furrows on bridge of nose	Wrinkling the nose	Pyramidalis
Crease from sides of nose to corners of mouth	Smiling	Risorius
Lines from corners of mouth to chin	Looking down in the mouth	Depressors of angles of the mouth
Vertical furrows on upper lip	Pursing the lips, tension, smoking, ill-fitting dentures	Orbicularis oris

Questions

1. Explain what is meant by the following terms:
   (a) the orbits;   (b) sinuses;   (c) crow's feet;   (d) expression lines.
2. Explain how:
   (a) contraction of a muscle may wrinkle the skin;
   (b) a dimple is formed in the skin.
3. What are the functions of the skull?
4. Give the names of the following:
   (a) two muscles of mastication;
   (b) two muscles in the neck;
   (c) two circular muscles in the face.
5. Name the muscle which causes:
   (a) vertical frown lines on the forehead;
   (b) horizontal lines across the forehead;
   (c) laughter lines round the eyes;
   (d) smiling.

Chapter 4

The skin

The purpose of make-up is to enhance the appearance of the facial area by the application of suitable cosmetic materials and at the same time to keep the skin in a soft and pliable condition. Skin varies in colour, texture and thickness from one person to another, and also in different areas of the body of any individual person. Considerable changes take place in the skin during ageing, particularly to the facial skin which is constantly exposed to variations in external conditions. In order to make accurate assessments of the needs of a client, a knowledge of the structure of the skin is a first essential.

The structure of the skin

The skin is shown in section in Fig. 4.1 and consists of two main layers.
1. **The epidermis** or scarf skin forms the outer layer.
2. **The dermis,** also called the corium or cutis vera (the true skin), forms the inner layer and constitutes the main bulk of the skin.

Below the dermis is a fatty *subcutaneous layer* which in most parts of the body, including the facial area, loosely connects the skin to the underlying muscle. The boundary between the epidermis and the dermis is clearly defined but the dermis merges gradually into the subcutaneous layer. The fat in this layer acts as insulation and helps to preserve body heat. It also acts as a cushion under the skin so providing a firm foundation.

The epidermis

The epidermis consists of five layers of cells though there are no sharp divisions between the layers. The outer layer of dead flat scaly cells made of a tough protein called keratin is constantly being rubbed away by friction and replaced by new cells produced by cell division in the lower living layer. A few nerve endings enter the lower epidermis but no blood vessels. The nutrients required by the living epidermal cells are carried by tissue fluid from the blood vessels in the dermis below. The thickness of the epidermis varies in different parts of the body, being thickest on the soles of the feet and palms of the hands, and thin in the face particu-

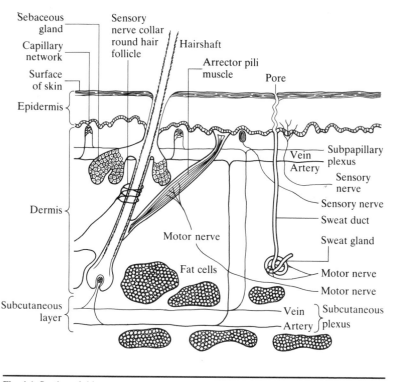

Fig. 4.1 Section of skin

larly in the eyelids and round the eyes. The thickness also varies in different races, usually being much thicker in dark-skinned people.

The layers of the epidermis are shown in Fig. 4.2. Starting with the lowest they are as follows:

The *stratum germinativum* (the germinating or basal cell layer) is a single layer of soft cuboid cells regularly arranged to form the junction with the dermis. These cells divide to form new cells which push the adjacent ones nearer to the skin surface. The germinating layer is continuous round the hair follicles, sebaceous glands and sweat glands, which may appear to be part of the dermis but are all formed by downgrowth of epidermal tissue into the dermis. The cells of this layer also divide to repair surface damage to the skin. Smaller cells called *melanocytes* are present among the basal cells and produce granules or melanosomes containing the yellow, brown or black pigment *melanin* which is the main colouring agent of the skin. In black skin a greater number of melanosomes are produced which are also of a larger size than those in white skin, though the actual number of melanocytes is about the same. Each melanocyte

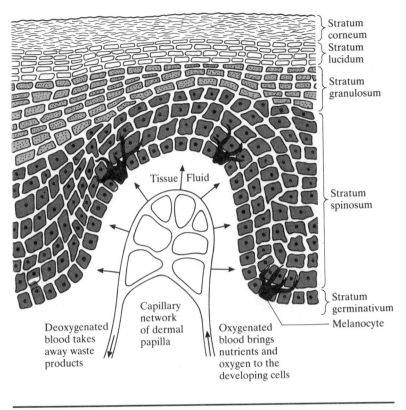

Stratum
corneum

Stratum
lucidum

Stratum
granulosum

Stratum
spinosum

Tissue Fluid

Stratum
germinativum

Melanocyte

Deoxygenated
blood takes
away waste
products

Capillary
network
of dermal
papilla

Oxygenated
blood brings
nutrients and
oxygen to the
developing cells

Fig. 4.2 The layers of the epidermis

has several dendrites (finger-like processes which protrude from the cell) through which the granules are distributed to the surrounding cells.

The *stratum spinosum* (the prickle cell layer) consists of a much deeper layer of cells than the germinating layer. Some of the cells have spiny outgrowths through which it is thought that melanin granules from the melanocytes enter the cells. As they travel through this layer the cells gradually become flatter. The prickle cell layer and the germinating layer together form the living part of the epidermis or the *malpighian layer*.

The *stratum granulosum* (the granular layer) is an area in which great changes take place in the cells. Here the nuclei of the cells begin to break down leading to the death of the cells, the spiny outgrowths become less distinct and the production of keratin starts by the formation of clear keratohyalin granules. The cells become harder and flatter. In white skins the destruction of melanin by enzymes also begins.

The *stratum lucidum* (the clear layer) is a very shallow layer in facial skin but is thick in the soles of the feet and the palms of the hands. The flattened cells of this layer are completely filled with keratin and have no nuclei. In white skins the destruction of melanin is completed here.

The *stratum corneum* (the horny or cornified layer) is the outer layer of the epidermis and consists of flat dead scales of keratin. Clumps of the scales are gradually desquamated or shed from the surface of the skin. In dark skins the horny layer is both thicker and tougher, and more desquamation takes place, sometimes giving the skin a slightly grey cast. Melanin is also still present in the horny layer and in the desquamated scales. Epidermal cells take about a month to travel from the germinating layer to the outer edge of the skin.

The dermis

The surface of the dermis is covered with tiny cone-shaped projections called *dermal papillae* which fit into corresponding hollows in the underside of the epidermis. The dermal papillae contain both nerve endings and networks of blood capillaries.

The dermis supports the epidermis and consists of a dense network of interwoven bundles of fibres embedded in a jelly-like ground substance. There are two types of fibres in the dermis (see Fig. 4.3):

1. *Collagen fibres* are present in the greater numbers and form a dense network, lying in layers parallel to the skin surface with alternate layers at right-angles to each other. Collagen is a protein consisting of non-elastic fibres arranged in a folded or wave-like structure. The amount of collagen in black skin is much greater than in white skin.
2. *Elastic fibres* are made of a protein called elastin. They lie between and run parallel to the collagen fibres. These fibres enable the skin to stretch as in pregnancy and to spring back when released. The stretching of the elastic fibres causes the unfolding of the collagen fibres but they normally return to their folded form as the elastic fibres relax.

The *ground substance* is which the fibres are embedded consists of a jelly-like substance called a proteoglycan (a compound of protein and sugars) capable of absorbing considerable amounts of water, so giving firmness to the skin, and acting like a cushion to resist compression by returning the skin to its original shape after being dented.

The dermis also contains several different types of cells which tend to be widely spaced throughout the ground substance.

1. *Mast cells* secrete histamine when the skin reacts to allergens or when the skin is damaged. Histamine causes dilation of the surrounding blood vessels so bringing extra blood to the area to aid repair.
2. *Phagocytic cells* are wandering white blood cells which are able to travel around the dermis destroying foreign matter and bacteria.
3. *Fibroblasts* are concerned with the secretion of proteoglycans for the ground substance of the dermis, and also play a part in the production of collagen fibres.

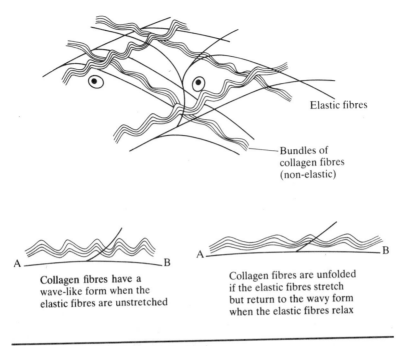

Elastic fibres

Bundles of
collagen fibres
(non-elastic)

Collagen fibres have a
wave-like form when the
elastic fibres are unstretched

Collagen fibres are unfolded
if the elastic fibres stretch
but return to the wavy form
when the elastic fibres relax

Fig. 4.3 Collagen and elastic fibres in the dermis

The blood supply to the skin

The dermis is well supplied with blood vessels to bring nutrients and
oxygen to the actively dividing cells of the epidermis to which there is no
direct blood supply, and also to enable the skin to play its part in the
regulation of body temperature. A network or plexus of arteries in the
subcutaneous layer or lower dermis runs parallel to the surface of the
skin (see Fig. 4.1). Smaller vessels leave the dermal plexus at right-
angles, extending towards the surface of the skin with branches leading
off to form capillary networks round the hair follicles, sweat glands and
sebaceous glands. These smaller vessels join to form another plexus, the
sub-papillary plexus, just below the dermal papillae. Branches from this
second plexus form capillary networks in the dermal papillae themselves.
De-oxygenated blood passes back through a series of small veins to the
main venous network of the skin in the lower dermis.

The amount of blood flowing near the surface of the skin is controlled
by nerve endings in the artery walls. If the body is overheating the small
arteries dilate, so increasing the blood supply to the skin, and more heat
is lost to the surrounding air. If the body is cooled the arteries become

constricted, less blood flows near the surface of the skin and therefore less heat is lost by the body. In this way the skin assists in maintenance of a constant body temperature. The blood in the skin also serves as a reservoir which may be diverted elsewhere in an emergency.

The nerves of the skin (see Fig. 4.1)

Most of the nerves in the skin are *sensory nerves*, that is they carry impulses from nerve endings in the skin to the brain. These nerve endings are sensitive to heat, cold, pain and pressure.

There are, however, a few *motor nerves* which carry impulses from the brain to the skin. These are responsible for the dilation and constriction of the blood vessels, the secretion of perspiration from the sweat glands, and the contraction of the arrector pili muscles attached to hair follicles. The arrector pili muscles contract in cold conditions or in states of fear. They make hairs stand erect in an attempt to trap an insulating layer of still air close to the skin surface to help to retain body heat, and also cause the skin at the mouth of the follicles to be raised in goose pimples.

The appendages of the skin

Hairs, the sebaceous glands, sweat glands and nails are known as the appendages of the skin. They are all formed from epidermal tissue which extends down into the dermis. Nails are considered separately in Chapter 16 in the section of the book concerning manicure.

Hair

Hairs grow by the division of cells at the base of minute pits in the skin called *hair follicles* (see Fig. 4.4). The stratum germinativum of the epidermis is continuous round the follicles, and it is from this layer that the hairs grow. The dermis projects upwards into the base of each follicle to form a *hair papilla* which contains blood capillaries bringing nourishment to the growing hair. The walls of the follicle are known as the *outer root sheath*. The follicle is supplied with a collar of sensory nerve fibres which respond to touch and to the movement of the hair.

As new cells are formed, the older cells are pushed along the follicle and undergo changes similar to those taking place in the epidermis of the skin. The cells change shape and become hardened by the formation of the tough protein, keratin. The cell nuclei are destroyed leading to the death of the cells. While in the follicle the hair is protected by the *inner root sheath* which grows up alongside the hair. The part of the hair projecting above the surface of the skin is called the *hair shaft* and unless it has been cut its tip or hair point is always pointed.

The hair shaft is arranged in three distinct cylindrical layers (see Fig. 4.5), the *cuticle* on the outside, then the *cortex* and finally the *medulla* in the centre. The cuticle consists of from seven to eleven layers of overlap-

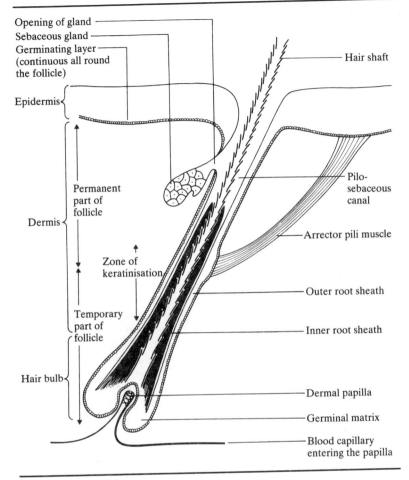

Opening of gland
Sebaceous gland
Germinating layer
(continuous all round
the follicle)

Epidermis

Hair shaft

Permanent
part of
follicle

Dermis

Pilo-
sebaceous
canal

Arrector pili muscle

Zone of
keratinisation

Outer root sheath

Temporary
part of
follicle

Inner root sheath

Hair bulb

Dermal papilla

Germinal matrix

Blood capillary
entering the papilla

Fig. 4.4 Hair and follicle

ping scales, the tips of which project towards the points of the hair. Immediately below the cuticle is the cortex which forms the main bulk of the hair, and consists of elongated cells containing a series of long keratinous fibres. Melanin, the colouring matter of hair, is also found in the cortex. The medulla or central core of the hair consists of a honeycomb of irregular areas of keratin with some air spaces between them. Unless the hair is particularly fine, a medulla is usually present in the coarse *terminal hairs* of the scalp, eyebrows and eyelashes, but not in the fine *lanugo hairs* of the foetus or in the fine downy *vellus hairs* which are found on most parts of the skin including the face.

A small muscle, the *arrector pili muscle*, extends from about one-third the way up the follicle to the underside of the epidermis. Nerve impulses

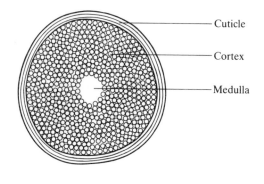

Fig. 4.5 Section of a hair shaft

carried from the brain by motor nerves cause contraction of the muscles in an attempt to make the hairs stand erect, and so trap an insulating layer of still air near the skin when the body is cold. The hairs of the eyebrows and eyelashes have no arrector pili muscles.

The growth of hair is not continuous since after a period of active growth known as *anagen*, a period of change (*catagen*) occurs during which the lower part of the follicle breaks down and the follicle becomes much shorter. This leads to a resting stage (*telogen*) during which there is no hair growth. The follicle then lengthens, a new hair begins to grow and the old hair is shed. About a hundred scalp hairs are shed in this way every day. Eyebrows and lashes also undergo these changes, so periodic shedding of these hairs takes place as well.

The sebaceous glands

Sebaceous glands are small sac-like pouches usually opening into hair follicles though large glands, frequently seen in the folds of the nose and often present in black skin, may open directly on to the surface of the skin. A sebaceous gland and its associated follicle are together known as a *pilo-sebaceous unit*. On the face, sebaceous glands are most numerous along the forehead and down the centre of the face, that is in the folds at the sides of the nostrils (the *naso-labial folds*) and on the chin. The glands continuously secrete an oily substance called *sebum*, the amount of secretion being controlled by hormones and not by nerves.

Sebum coats both the surface of the skin and the hair. The coating on the skin keeps the epidermis supple by preventing evaporation of water from the horny layer. It also prevents excessive absorption of water from the outside, which could cause swelling of the epidermis. Sebum has slight antiseptic and fungicidal properties. Consideration of the amount of sebum produced by the skin is important in deciding the correct treatment and choice of cosmetics for a particular client.

The sweat glands

There are two types of sweat glands in the skin, the eccrine glands and the apocrine glands.

Eccrine sweat glands or sudoriferous glands (see Fig. 4.6) are present in all parts of the skin though they are most numerous in the soles of the feet and in the palms of the hands. The glands consist of a coiled tube lying in the dermis, with a long duct which is straight at first but which takes a spiral course through the epidermis to open in a pore on the surface of the skin. The sweat secreted by the gland is a clear liquid containing 98 per cent water with about 2 per cent sodium chloride (common salt) and traces of many other substances including urea and lactic acid. The secretion of sweat is increased by heat and nervous tension and is under the control of motor nerves.

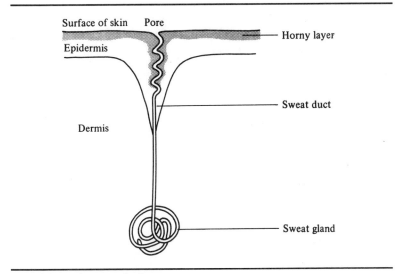

Fig. 4.6 An eccrine sweat gland

The main function of sweat is to help to maintain constant body temperature. The evaporation of sweat from the surface of the skin requires heat which is taken from the skin so cooling the body. In temperate climates about one litre of sweat per day evaporates from the skin without it becoming wet. This continual sweating is known as *insensible perspiration*. Sweat also helps to maintain the horny layer in a pliable state by keeping the keratin moist. A very minor function of sweat is to rid the body of waste products such as urea and lactic acid.

Apocrine sweat glands (see Fig. 4.7) are usually larger than eccrine glands and are limited to certain areas of the body such as the axillae (armpits) and the pubic region. Each gland consists of a coiled tube with a narrow duct opening into a hair follicle just above the level of the sebaceous gland. Development of these glands takes place only at puberty, the secretion being controlled by hormones as well as by nerves. The secretion is a milky fluid containing fat particles. The breakdown of this type of sweat by bacteria on the surface of the skin leads to unpleasant body odour.

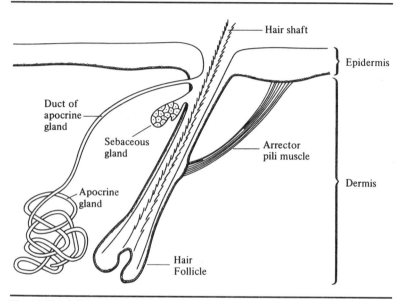

Fig. 4.7 Hair follicle with apocrine gland

Skin types

Basically there are four skin types, each of which requires different cosmetic treatment.
1. *Normal skin.* It is quite rare for a client to have a normal skin. This type of skin is firm, of an even texture, usually blemish free and radiating a healthy pink glow. It is never shiny or dull and is neither too oily nor too dry. Normal skin is usually synonymous with young skin.
2. *Oily skin.* Also referred to as greasy skin, the excessive grease can be the result of over-active sebaceous glands, a diet containing too many fats and oils, or neglect in cleansing. This skin may appear sallow and shiny and have open pores; blackheads and spots are common and the skin is subject to acne. Oily skin is quite prevalent in teenagers.

3. *Dry skin.* This type of skin can appear flaky and has a tendency to feel tight after washing. It is often fine and sensitive so is readily irritated and reddens easily. Broken capillaries and milia are often found in this skin type. The lack of moisture and natural oils hastens the ageing process, so this skin may wrinkle prematurely, especially round the eyes. The excessive use of harsh soaps and skin toners together with over-exposure to the sun and the drying effect of low humidity in centrally heated rooms may be contributory factors to dry skin.

4. *Combination skin.* As its name suggests, this is a combination of two skin types: (a) oily and (b) dry. Invariably the greasy panel will be across the forehead and down the centre of the face affecting the nose and chin. The remaining areas, that is the skin around the eyes and on the cheeks, will be dry. This is the commonest skin type.

The colour of the skin

There is a wide variation of skin colour throughout the races of the world. African skins may vary from light brown through dark brown to black, which may have undertones of grey, red or yellow. Asian skins may be various shades of brown and include oriental skins, the yellowish skins of the Chinese and the more creamy skins of the Japanese. European skins vary from the more sallow skins of southern areas to the much fairer skins of the north.

The final colour of skin depends on several factors:

1. The amount and type of melanin produced by the melanocytes. This may be increased by exposure to ultra-violet rays either from the sun or from ultra-violet lamps.

2. The amount of melanin removed by enzyme action as the cells travel through the epidermis. Again this may be affected by exposure to ultra-violet rays which tend to prevent the breakdown of melanin and cause it to darken.

3. The natural yellowish colour (carotene) of the epidermal cells themselves. This factor ceases to be important if a large amount of melanin is present.

4. The amount of blood flowing through the capillaries of the upper dermis. If the blood vessels are dilated, the skin becomes red due to oxyhaemoglobin in the red blood cells. If the blood vessels are constricted by cold, the blood flow is slower and the presence of de-oxygenated blood makes the skin blue. Again this factor depends on the amount of melanin in the skin. The darker the skin the less obvious is the effect of changes in blood supply.

The functions of the skin

The skin may be regarded as one of the major organs of the body and has many important functions.

1. *Protection.* The skin provides a waterproof coat which protects the body from dirt, minor injuries, bacterial invasion and chemical attack. The first barrier is the layer of sebum and sweat produced by the skin and forming a slightly acid film over its surface. This is sometimes known as the *acid mantle.* The acidity (pH of 4.5 – 6) discourages the growth of bacteria. Sebum is also slightly fungicidal so helps to prevent fungal growth in the skin. The second barrier is the stratum corneum which acts as a filter against invading bacteria. Any organisms passing through this barrier may be attacked by wandering phagocytic cells in the dermis. Melanin protects the underlying tissues from damage by ultra-violet rays in sunlight.
2. *The regulation of body temperature.* The skin helps to keep body temperature constant at 36.9 °C by the dilation or constriction of blood vessels near the surface, the cooling effect of the evaporation of sweat and the insulating properties of subcutaneous fat.
3. *As a sense organ.* The skin acts as a sense organ to detect changes in temperature and pressure and to register pain. It thus informs the brain of changes in the environment.
4. *Vitamin D production* The action of ultra-violet rays on sterols in the epidermis results in the formation of vitamin D.
5. *Storage.* The skin acts as a storage depot for fat and water and also as a reservoir for blood which can be diverted to other organs as required.
6. *Excretion.* Waste products such as lactic acid and urea are secreted in sweat though this is a very minor function of the skin.

Questions

1. What is the function in the skin of each of the following:
   (a) melanin;   (b) the stratum corneum;   (c) eccrine sweat glands;   (d) phagocytic cells in the dermis?
2 Describe the changes which take place in the cells of the epidermis as they travel from the basal layer to the surface of the skin.
3. What is meant by each of the following:
   (a) the acid mantle of the skin;
   (b) a pilo-sebaceous unit;
   (c) the naso-labial fold;
   (d) the appendages of the skin?
4. Explain the difference between the following:
   (a) a sensory nerve and a motor nerve;
   (b) anagen and telogen;
   (c) eccrine and apocrine sweat glands;
   (d) collagen fibres and elastic fibres in the dermis.
5. Discuss the causes of (a) greasy skin and (b) dry skin. Describe the characteristic blemishes of each.

Chapter 5

The condition of facial skin

Skin condition depends on the state of both the epidermis and the dermis. It may be affected by external influences such as exposure to the sun's rays, the humidity of the surrounding air and the application of cosmetics, as well as by internal factors including the water content of the skin, the secretion of sebum and sweat, diet and general health. The state of the skin also changes gradually during the ageing process.

The water balance of the skin

To be soft and pliable the stratum corneum must contain at least 10 per cent by weight of water. If the layer is dehydrated and the water content falls below this level, flexibility is lost and the epidermis becomes hard and brittle with a tendency to crack. In addition to the moisture lost as sweat from the pores of the skin, a smaller amount is continually lost from the surface of the stratum corneum. Unless this surface loss is prevented or is replaced by moisture from the lower epidermis and the dermis below, dehydration will take place.

The amount of moisture in the stratum corneum depends on the following factors (see Fig.5.1):

1. *The humidity of the surrounding air.* In conditions of very high humidity the skin may become waterlogged since evaporation of moisture from the surface is prevented. At average humidity the loss from the skin is usually fully replaced by the passage of moisture upwards from the lower epidermis and the dermis. If, however, the humidity is very low, as is often the case in centrally heated rooms and on cold dry winter days, loss of moisture may be greater than that gained from below and dehydration occurs.

2. *The water-holding capacity of the skin.* The amount of water which the stratum corneum is capable of holding is reduced by continual degreasing and is also lowered during the ageing process. In addition, ageing reduces the store of water held in the ground substance of the dermis so less water is available to replace any epidermal loss. In old age the skin may thus suffer considerable dehydration.

3. *The amount of oily material on the skin surface.* A layer of oil on the surface of the skin tends to stop the loss of water from the stratum corneum. The oil is said to form an *occlusive* layer which enables

water to build up from below, and keeps the surface layer of the skin supple. If an adequate amount of sebum is produced by the sebaceous glands, this acts as an *emollient* or skin softener, since the oily sebum delays water loss. An insufficiency of sebum may be counteracted by the application of oil to the skin. Cosmetic creams and lotions in the form of emulsions containing both oil and water are particularly effective emollients, since the water content directly softens the stratum corneum and the oil content tends to stop water loss. The emollient action of such emulsions is often increased by the addition of *humectants* such as glycerol and sorbitol, which attract water to themselves from the atmosphere so bringing extra water to the skin surface.

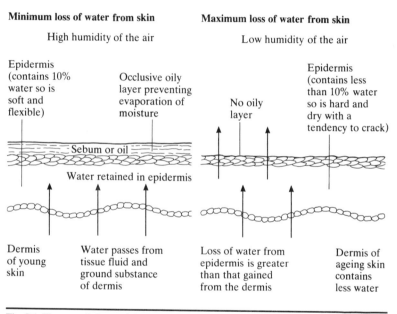

Minimum loss of water from skin

High humidity of the air

Epidermis (contains 10% water so is soft and flexible)

Occlusive oily layer preventing evaporation of moisture

Sebum or oil

Water retained in epidermis

Dermis of young skin

Water passes from tissue fluid and ground substance of dermis

Maximum loss of water from skin

Low humidity of the air

Epidermis (contains less than 10% water so is hard and dry with a tendency to crack)

No oily layer

Loss of water from epidermis is greater than that gained from the dermis

Dermis of ageing skin contains less water

Fig. 5.1 The water balance of the skin

The structure of emulsions

An emulsion consists of minute droplets of one liquid suspended in another liquid. The two liquids concerned must be insoluble in each other. All emulsions thus consist of two phases, the droplets form the *disperse phase* and the liquid in which the droplets are suspended forms the *continuous phase*. Most common emulsions are mixtures of oil and water. Droplets of oil suspended in water form an *oil-in-water* emulsion, and droplets of water suspended in oil form a *water-in-oil* emulsion (see Fig. 5.2). To prevent the separation of the oil and water of an emulsion into two distinct layers, a third substance called an *emulsifying agent* or emulsifyer must be added to make the emulsion more permanent. Various substances such as soap and soapless detergents, cetyl alcohol and lanolin will act as emulsifying agents by surrounding the droplets of the disperse phase, so preventing them from coming together to form a separate layer. The droplets in an emulsion are large enough to be seen through a microscope and such emulsions take the form of creams or milky liquids.

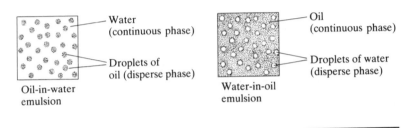

Fig. 5.2 Structure of emulsions

Substances often used in the oil phase of cosmetic emulsions include the following:
1. *Vegetable oils* obtained from plants, e.g. almond oil and olive oil.
2. *Mineral oils* which are derived from petroleum obtained from the ground. In addition to gases which are used for heating purposes and petrol used in car engines, petroleum products include mineral oils, petroleum jelly and paraffin wax, all of which may be used in the oil phase of emulsions.

   In cosmetics, mineral oils are often preferred to vegetable oils since they are better grease solvents, are less likely to become rancid or contaminated with micro-organisms, and are less viscous and sticky. However, mineral oil used by itself is a good solvent for sebum and tends to be too degreasing for dry skin. Products for use on dry skin thus always contain at least a small proportion of vegetable oil in addition to mineral oil.
3. *Stearic acid* which is a white waxy solid. This forms a very light cream which is not as greasy as vegetable or mineral oils. On the skin it remains as a matt non-greasy layer of minute crystals which do not melt at skin temperature.
4. *Lanolin* which is obtained from sheep's wool and is similar to sebum. This is often added to mineral oils since it is an excellent emollient. It is, however, a known sensitiser and its presence in any product must always be stated on the label.
5. *Isopropyl myristate*, an oily liquid often added to mineral or vegetable oil in small quantities to reduce the greasiness of a product.

6. *Waxes* such as *ozokerite* and *ceresin* are used to thicken the oil phase and reduce the greasiness of the product by absorbing oil. Ozokerite is mined from the ground and is known as an earth wax. When refined, it is a hard white solid of minute crystals, so is said to have a micro-crystalline structure. Ceresin is made by purifying ozokerite.

The properties of emulsions and their effect on the skin

The two types of emulsion have different properties and have different effects on skin.

1. Oil-in-water emulsions (see Fig. 5.3)
Oil-in-water (O/W) emulsions may be diluted with water and can be washed from the skin using water alone. The water phase is often thickened by adding gums or polyvinyl pyrrolidone (a plastic resin).

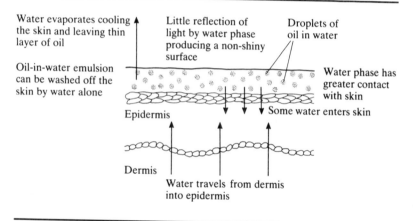

Fig. 5.3 Oil-in-water emulsion on the skin

This type of emulsion is used in day creams, e.g. moisturising creams and foundation creams, for the following reasons:

(a) Since the continuous phase is the water phase, water has a greater contact with the skin than oil. Some of this water may be absorbed by the skin, giving an immediate moisturising effect. This effect is heightened if humectants are added to the water phase to attract more water to the product.

(b) They produce lighter creams than water-in-oil emulsions since the proportion of oil is usually lower, and leave a very thin emollient layer of oil on the skin when the water has evaporated.

(c) They reflect less light than water-in-oil emulsions since the oil, which is more reflective than water, is enclosed in the water phase. A shiny appearance, which is undesirable in a day cream, is therefore avoided.

(d) They feel cool on the skin due to the evaporation of the water phase.
2. *Water-in-oil emulsions* (see Fig. 5.4)
Water-in-oil (W/O) emulsions do not mix easily with water and cannot be washed off the skin by water alone. They must either be wiped off with a tissue, or removed by use of a detergent or a fat-solvent. They have little cooling effect since the water content evaporates slowly.

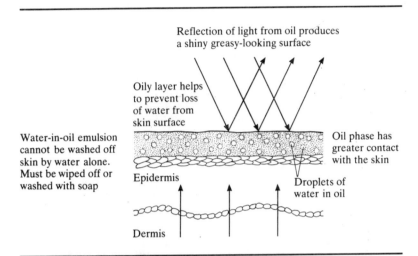

Fig. 5.4 Water-in-oil emulsion on the skin

These emulsions are mainly used for night creams, massage creams and cleansing creams, for the following reasons:
(a) They are more lubricant and occlusive, since the oil phase has the greater contact with the skin.
(b) They are usually thicker and greasier than oil-in-water emulsions since the oil content is higher.
(c) Their highly reflective and shiny appearance is unimportant in night creams and in creams which are left on the skin for a short time only.
To have a moisturising and emollient effect on the skin, so improving skin condition, cosmetic emulsions must be left on for some time. Thus moisturising creams and night creams are more beneficial as conditioners than massage creams or cleansing creams which have only a short contact time on the skin.

Absorption of substances by the skin

Some cosmetic creams, particularly night creams, often have added ingredients which are designed to improve skin condition by being absorbed into the skin. Since the function of the epidermis is to protect the body by preventing such penetration, the absorption is necessarily limited. Some fatty substances are known to reach the dermis via the hair follicles and sebaceous glands. These include vitamin A and oestrogen, a female sex hormone. However, the amount of vitamin A absorbed would be very small compared to the amount normally taken orally. Oestrogen creams are thought to be effective in delaying ageing by restoring the water retention properties of the skin. The use of creams for this purpose would have to be continuous and there is a danger of unwanted side effects.

Effect of diet on the skin

In western society the main nutrients (proteins, fats and carbohydrates) are unlikely to be lacking in the normal diet. However, drastic reducing diets may deplete the subcutaneous fat causing the facial skin of even a young person to become baggy and the cheeks hollow. Some dehydration of the tissues may also occur, increasing the possibility of premature wrinkling. Excessive intake of alcohol may cause dehydration, as well as dilating the blood capillaries of the face and possibly leading to permanently dilated or 'broken' capillaries. Certain vitamins and minerals may be lacking in some diets. The vitamins and minerals most affecting the skin are listed in Table 5.1.

Table 5.1 Vitamins and minerals affecting the skin

Nutrient	Foods providing a good source	Effect on skin of deficiency in diet
Retinol (Vitamin A)	Dairy foods, liver, margarine, carrots, fish liver oils	Blockage of sweat and tear ducts by keratin. Plugs of keratin in follicles of upper arms and legs
Riboflavin (Vitamin B$_2$)	Milk, eggs, liver, kidney	Cracking of corners of mouth, fissuring of lips, seborrhoeic accumulations round the eyes and nose
Niacin (nicotinic acid) (a B group vitamin)	Meat, pulses, whole grain cereals	Type of dermatitis causing erythema as a symmetrical rash on face and neck with rough and scaly skin
Ascorbic acid (Vitamin C)	Citrus fruits, green vegetables, blackcurrants	Small haemorrhages round hair follicles, delay in healing wounds, breakdown of connective tissue, easy bruising
Iron	Liver, egg yolk, green vegetables	Paleness of the skin (due to anaemia)

The effect of ultra-violet rays on skin

Ultra-violet (UV) rays are present in sunlight but may also be produced by mercury vapour lamps. Many salons offer ultra-violet treatment to produce skin tanning; it is also useful for the treatment of psoriasis and acne. Ultra-violet rays travel in the form of waves. Along with the visible light rays and infra-red rays found in sunlight, and also radio waves, micro-waves and X-rays, they form a series of energy waves known as electromagnetic waves. All these forms of radiation differ from each other because they have different wavelengths, a wavelength being the distance between two adjacent wave crests of a wave train (see Fig. 5.5).

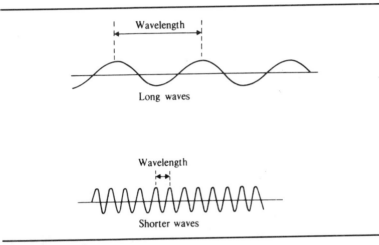

Fig. 5.5 Wavelength

A classification of electromagnetic waves according to wavelength is shown in Table 5.2

Table 5.2 Electromagnetic waves

Type of wave	Wavelength	Uses
Radio waves	Long	Radio transmission
Television waves		Television transmission
Microwaves	Decreasing	Cooking
Infra-red		Heat treatments
Visible light		For sight; photography
Ultra-violet		Sun-ray treatment
X-rays	Very short	X-ray photography

Ultra-violet rays thus lie in the electromagnetic series between X-rays and visible light rays. They themselves are invisible rays with wavelengths between 200–400 nanometres, a nanometre (nm) being a thousand millionth of a metre. For treatment purposes, UV rays are subdivided into three groups, UVA, UVB and UVC, again according to wavelength (see Fig. 5.6).

UVC is never used for skin treatments but, since it is the most potent of the ultra-violet rays in destroying bacteria, it may be used in salon

Infra-red rays	Visible light	Ultra-violet rays			X-rays
		UVA	UVB	UVC	

700 nm	400 nm 320 nm 290 nm 200 nm	
Wavelength in nanometres	Wavelength decreasing	

Fig. 5.6 Wavelength of ultra-violet rays

'sterilising' cabinets where it is produced by mercury vapour lamps. The UVC from the sun is mostly absorbed in the upper atmosphere so does not reach the earth in sunlight.

The effect of exposure of the skin to ultra-violet rays is summarised in Table 5.3.

Table 5.3 Effect of exposure of the skin to ultra-violet radiation

Type of UV	Depth of skin penetration	Effect of moderate exposure	Effect of over-exposure
UVA	Through the epidermis and into dermis	Immediate but short-lived tan by darkening the melanin already in the skin	Erythema may occur after very prolonged exposure. Frequent over-use may cause ageing by damage to elastic fibres in dermis. Cataract (clouding of the lens of the eye) unless protective goggles are worn
UVB	To lower epidermis only	Delayed but long-lasting tan due to production of more melanin by melanocytes. Produces vitamin D in skin	Slight over-exposure: erythema appearing several hours later lasting 3–4 days. Longer over-exposure: burning and blistering of the skin. Repeated over-exposure: ageing and thickening of the skin, and possibly skin cancer. Cataract
UVC	To upper epidermis only	Not used for skin treatment (used in UV Cabinets)	Not produced by the UV lamps used for skin tanning

Apparatus used for suntanning

Two types of apparatus are available to produce suntan artificially.
1. *Sun lamps* are high-pressure mercury vapour lamps which produce UVA, UVB and UVC, the latter being absorbed by a special glass filter surrounding the lamp so leaving just the UVA and UVB. This type of radiation is thus similar to that produced by the sun. Contact time must be short to avoid over-exposure and possible burning, while the tan itself is delayed and long-lasting.
2. *Sun beds* are a safer and more popular alternative to sun lamps. Low-pressure mercury vapour lamps similar to fluorescent light tubes pro-duce UVC which then strikes a chemical substance (known as a phos-

phor) lining the inside of the tube which converts the UVC to visible light and UVA only. Sun beds contain a series of these tubes as shown in Fig. 5.7. The tan produced is immediate and temporary, lasting only a few days. Some types of sun bed lamps also produce a little UVB to increase melanin production and encourage a more lasting tan. The effect of tanning builds up gradually over a series of treatments. Once a tan is acquired the skin is protected from erythema and burning.

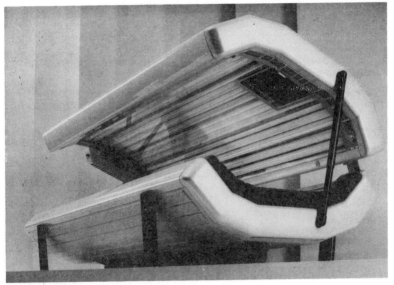

Fig. 5.7 Sun bed

Precautions in the use of ultra-violet rays

1. UV rays are damaging to the eyes and protective goggles should always be worn even for sun bed treatments. Contact lenses should be removed.
2. Careful attention should be paid to manufacturers' instructions for sun beds and lamps to avoid the possibility of over-exposing the client resulting in erythema, peeling or blistering. Sun bed sessions should be increased gradually, starting with 15 minutes and rising to a maximum of 30 minutes taken at not more than 2–3 day intervals. Too frequent exposure to UV may cause premature ageing of the skin and thickening of the epidermis.
3. The client's make-up and perfume should be removed as certain chemicals included in cosmetics may increase the effect of UV, producing painful erythema. This effect is known as photosensitivity.
4. The client's hair should be covered, especially if bleached, tinted or permed. UV tends to bleach hair and relax perms.

5. Accurate records of client exposure times and reactions should be kept.

Contra-indications to the use of UV

1. Use of UV is not recommended for clients with sensitive or very fair skins which do not tan easily, since these skins readily burn.
2. Some people react to UV with severe itching of the skin, dermatitis or with nausea and headaches. UV should be avoided by those who regularly suffer from headaches or migraine.
3. Exposure should also be avoided by clients with skin complaints other than psoriasis and acne, especially sufferers from eczema and dermatitis and those who are subject to repeated cold sores.
4. Certain drugs cause photosensitivity and people taking tranquillisers, antibiotics and anti-diabetic tablets should avoid UV.
5. UV should be avoided during pregnancy, and by people with heart conditions, diabetes and either high or low blood pressure.

The weathering of the skin

Weathering, that is exposure to the sun and wind, is the commonest cause of premature ageing and lining of the skin. Ultra-violet rays in sunlight cause degeneration of dermal elastic fibres resulting in wrinkling, thickening of the epidermis by increasing the rate of cell division in the stratum germinativum, possible burning of the tissues, and irregular pigmentation such as lentigines or age spots. Exposure to cold winds may produce excessive drying of the skin with cracking or chapping of the epidermis; broken capillaries may also develop. General over-exposure to the weather leads to a leathery, deeply wrinkled skin.

The easy availability of world travel aggravates the problem of weathering. Hot dry desert conditions produce both sun damage and dryness of the skin. Tropical climates may also result in sun damage, but the high humidity of these areas may in addition produce greasy coarse skin. Cold dry arctic climates cause excessive dryness and the circulation of the blood may be drastically reduced leading to frostbite. For white skins a temperate climate is kindest, dark-skinned people being much less affected by the sun's rays. A gradually tanned skin can, however, withstand exposure to the sun better. The damaging effects of excessive sunshine may be minimised by shading the face with a broad-brimmed hat and using sun screen creams. Drying conditions may be combated by increased use of moisturisers and skin conditioning night creams.

The ageing of the skin

Ageing of skin takes place gradually but continuously throughout life but is first noticeable by the appearance of wrinkles and lines particularly around the eyes and mouth. This is largely due to damage to the elastic fibres in the dermis by the sun's ultra-violet rays. Areas of the skin such as the face and hands, which are constantly exposed to the sun, age more rapidly than areas normally kept covered. Black skin is better protected against sun damage since melanin, which is present in larger quantities, absorbs ultra-violet rays allowing fewer to reach the dermis. Degeneration of elastic fibres is thus delayed and the skin stays firm longer. For this reason the ageing of black skin rarely starts until about the age of 60 years. The bone structure of black races also often assists in delaying ageing since their high cheek bones and a more protruding jawlines help to retain the shape of the skin.

Other important factors affecting ageing include the gradual reduction of the blood supply to the skin, which results in a decrease in the renewal rate of cells and consequent thinning of the skin, a lowering of the water-holding capacity of the ground substance of the dermis causing the skin to become flabby, soft and loose, and changes in pigmentation.

The time scale of the ageing of the face

Although the signs of ageing vary considerably in the faces of different people, each decade produces its own characteristic features.

The teenage years

An increase in hormone production at puberty leads to enlargement of the sebaceous glands and excessive production of sebum. The teenage skin may thus be prone to blemishes, e.g. spots or acne, due to excessive oiliness. Otherwise the youthful skin is firm, smooth and shows no sign of age lines or wrinkles.

The blooming years

This is the age from 20–30 years when the face is well defined, has lost any trace of teenage plumpness and problems of hormone imbalance. The skin is both healthy and in prime condition. Slight traces of ageing will begin towards the end of this period as degeneration begins in the elastic fibres of the dermis. This takes the form of very fine lines, particularly round the eyes where the skin is thin and there is little supporting subcutaneous fat.

The waning years

The true onset of the ageing process takes place between the ages of 30–40 years. Expression lines such as crow's feet and frown marks are the first type of permanent wrinkling to appear during ageing. These result from the repeated contraction of the muscles of facial expression below the surface of the skin of the face. Skin colour, texture and condition also start to wane during this period.

The middle years

These are the years from 40–50. Broken capillaries may appear in the skin which now begins to look more delicate. Elasticity continues to decrease and the skin develops a baggy appearance. In young tissue, collagen fibres are gradually replaced by new fibres, but the amount of skin collagen decreases from early adulthood onwards so lessening the support for the epidermis. Elastic fibres normally keep the collagen fibres in their wavy form except when the skin is stretched. When the elastic fibres degenerate, the collagen fibres are no longer pulled back so the skin starts to sag and the contours drop. Due to the occurrence of the menopause during these years, hormonal imbalance may result in the appearance of adolescent-type problem skin and enlarged pores become a common feature. Hot flushes may also occur at this time.

The declining years

During the years from 50–60 the skin may become coarse but is thin and papery. Several factors contribute to this thinning. The dermal papillae become flattened, there is loss of subcutaneous fat and a lower rate of cell division in the stratum germinativum due to gradual reduction in blood supply. Lines and wrinkles now become apparent all over the skin though these are relatively shallow.

The skin may also appear to be extremely loose, partly due to continued degeneration of elastic and collagen fibres, but also due to a reduction in the water-holding capacity of the ground substance of the dermis which acts as a cushion to keep the skin firm. Consequently the skin collapses with dropped contours at the jawline, the possible development of a double chin and baggy skin under the eyes. Dryness is now a common feature. Hirsuitism, the growth of facial hair by a female, may cause distress if terminal hair replaces vellus hair in the lip and mouth area.

The latter years

From the age of 60 the secretion of sebum is reduced, especially in females, leading to further drying of the skin since sebum acts by preventing the evaporation of moisture from the epidermis. Thinning of the skin may also increase due to further decline of fatty tissue. Pigmentation may change dramatically. The number of melanocytes decreases and they become less active. Mottling of the skin sometimes results when some of the epidermal cells lose contact with the melanocytes. Sometimes melanin becomes concentrated in certain areas to produce brown patches or age spots, which increase in size on exposure to the sun. The fine lines and wrinkling of the skin surface increase, especially in the neck area which often becomes very crêpey; skin tags may also appear on the neck. Sluggish blood circulation causes the skin to lose its normal pink colour and become more sallow; it may also feel cold to the touch. The area round the eyes is often dark and puffy.

The prevention of premature ageing

Very fine lines may be reduced by keeping the skin well hydrated by adequate moisturising. Deep lines can only be treated by cosmetic camouflage using concealer creams to level out the skin.

Precautions to help prevent premature ageing
1. Avoid over-exposure to the sun and wind.
2. Maintain a high level of general health:
    (a) by ensuring an adequate and well-balanced diet (in particular, avoid excessive slimming diets);
    (b) by taking a reasonable amount of exercise in the fresh air;
    (c) by avoiding stress, overwork and lack of sleep.
3. Avoid cosmetic neglect of the skin by using moisturiser and night creams regularly.
4. Avoid excessive facial expression such as frowning, raising the eyebrows, and screwing up the eyes when smoking or in bright sunlight or through neglecting to wear spectacles if these are required.

Questions

1. In what positions on the face are expression lines usually found? Explain why such lines appear on the ageing face.
2. What is meant by the following:
    (a) an emollient;   (b) a humectant;   (c) weathering of the skin;   (d) an oil-in-water emulsion?
3. Explain why black skin normally ages more slowly than white skin.
4. What advice would you give to a client who requested very frequent sun bed treatment?
5. Discuss the effect on the skin of each of the following:
    (a) ultra-violet radiation;   (b) a drastic slimming diet;   (c) excessive consumption of alcohol;   (d) lack of sleep.

Chapter 6

Skin disorders

One of the objects of make-up is to disguise minor blemishes or imperfections of the skin. It is important therefore that the cosmetician should be aware of the different types of blemish, their causes and their treatment. The ability to distinguish between those it is safe to cover, those which are contra-indicative of treatment and those requiring medical attention is most important.

Blemishes may be present as a result of some congenital malformation, an abnormal functioning of the skin, infection by micro-organisms or damage by an external agent such as the sun, chemical or physical trauma. Often a *predisposing* or *contributing factor* may be present making a person more susceptible to a particular condition or disease at a particular time. For instance, damage by cuts or abrasions is a predisposing factor to the entry of bacteria into the skin and the development of boils or impetigo; the increased secretion of sebum at puberty is a predisposing factor to the development of acne.

The various types of blemish or *lesions* which may occur are listed below and illustrated in diagrammatic section in Fig. 6.1.

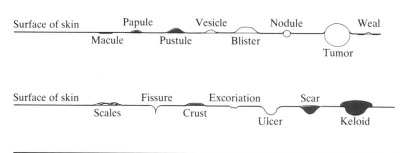

Fig. 6.1 Types of lesion

A macule is a small abnormally coloured area of skin which is level with the skin's surface so may be seen but not felt, e.g. a freckle. The macule may be darker or lighter than the surrounding skin.

A papule is a small, solid, raised area of unbroken skin which often develops into a pustule.

A pustule consists of a small collection of pus which is visible through a raised portion of the epidermis.

A vesicle is a small blister raised above the skin's surface and containing serum (a pale yellow liquid similar to blood plasma). Vesicles usually disappear without forming a scar.

A bulla is a blister more than 0.5 cm in diameter and is similar to a vesicle but larger.

A nodule or **cyst** is a small rounded swelling which extends both above and below the surface of the skin.

A tumor is a swelling of the skin larger than a nodule, consisting of hard or soft tissue.

A weal (wheal) is a white raised area of skin containing fluid and surrounded by a red area. A weal may appear and disappear quite quickly, e.g. urticaria (hives).

A bruise is an area of unbroken skin discoloured by blood from damaged blood vessels in the dermis.

Scales are flakes of easily detached keratin, e.g. scales of dry skin or of psoriasis.

Fissures are cracks in the epidermis exposing the dermis.

A crust (scab) results from the drying out of fluid from a lesion, e.g. serum forms honey-coloured crusts, blood forms brown crusts.

An excoriation (an abrasion or scratch) results from the removal of the epidermis by friction.

An ulcer is an open sore involving both the dermis and epidermis. Healing is followed by scar formation.

A scar is the replacement tissue formed during the healing of a wound.

A keloid is an overgrown scar caused by over-development of connective tissue (collagen), and occurs most often in black skin.

Other effects of skin diseases and conditions include:

Erythema or areas of redness of the skin due to dilation of blood capillaries in the dermis. Erythema is not easily noticeable in black skin but appears as dark purple areas which are darker than the skin itself.

Hyperaemia means an increased blood flow to an area and often results in erythema.

Weeping is a continuous watery discharge from an area of broken skin.

Oedema is the swelling of tissues due to an accumulation of fluid.

Inflammation of skin tissue is due to an increase in the blood supply to an infected area of the skin, and may be accompanied by redness, swelling, pain and heat. The blood vessels dilate, causing erythema and an increase of temperature in the area. The invading bacteria are attacked by white blood cells, some of which may be killed along with the bacteria, resulting in the formation of a core of pus or a 'head' through which pus is eventually discharged. Epidermal cells (basal cells) multiply to repair the surface of the skin but a scar may result if the dermis has been damaged.

Skin infections caused by bacteria

Bacteria are minute single-celled organisms which may be identified by microscopic examination and classified according to shape. Cocci are small round bacteria which may be arranged in bunches (staphylococci) or in long chains (streptococci). Bacilli are rod-shaped and spirocheates have a spiral shape. Large numbers of bacteria inhabit the surface of the skin but many are harmless or non-pathogenic. The pathogens which are responsible for skin infections are mostly streptococci and staphylococci, and these may cause disease if they enter hair follicles or broken skin. The most common bacterial infections of the skin are boils, carbuncles and impetigo.

Boils (furuncles)

A boil is a deep abscess formed in a hair follicle due to staphylococcal infection. It begins as a tender inflamed papule which rapidly develops into a painful pustule. Pus is later discharged from the 'head' of the boil. Removal of the core of pus leaves a cavity which heals with a scar. Predisposing factors are poor general health, chronic illnesses such as diabetes, and the rubbing of the skin, especially at the back of the neck by the pressure of a collar. Boils should be treated by frequent local heat. No cosmetics should be applied to the infected area, and contact with the area should be avoided.

Carbuncles

A carbuncle is formed when several adjacent follicles are simultaneously infected by staphylococci and is in effect a group of boils which develop several 'heads'. Severe inflammation of the surrounding area of skin occurs and medical advice should be sought. No cosmetics should be applied to the affected area.

Impetigo

Impetigo (see Fig. 6.2) is a rapidly spreading bacterial infection of the surface of the skin. Staphylococci and streptococci are usually both present. The infection starts with red macules which quickly form small vesicles filled with serum. These later become typical honey-coloured crusts which are easily removed leaving areas of moist pink skin. Impetigo is often seen in children and is very contagious. The areas round the nose and mouth are most usually affected. Medical attention is required and treatment is usually by antibiotic creams.

Conjunctivitis (commonly called 'pink eye')

This is inflammation of the conjunctiva, the very thin skin covering the inner eyelid and the front of the eyeball. The condition is caused by

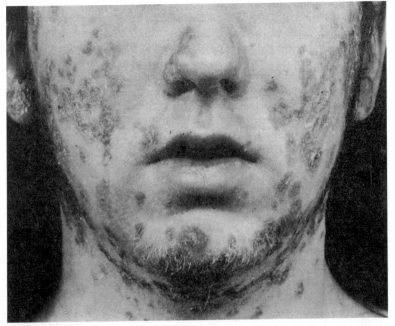

Fig. 6.2 Impetigo

bacterial infection following irritation of the conjunctiva by grit or powders, e.g. eye cosmetics entering the eye. Infected eyes look very red and
sore. Some pus may be formed and the condition is highly infectious. It is
readily passed from person to person by cross-infection from such objects
as infected towels. Treatment is by antibiotic lotions. No cosmetics
should be applied to the eye area and powdered cosmetics should be
avoided.

Skin infections caused by viruses

Viruses are very much smaller than bacteria and can only be seen by use
of an electron microscope. Viruses multiply inside living cells, then break
down the cell walls liberating the viruses to attack other cells. Since the
upper layers of the epidermis are dead tissue, viruses cannot live in these
areas or on the surface of the skin. They often, however, stay for a
considerable time in the lower epidermis, e.g. the virus causing recurrent
cold sores. Skin infections caused by viruses include warts, cold sores and
shingles.

Verrucae (warts)

A virus infection of the germinating layer of the epidermis causes a rapid
increase in the number of cells in the stratum spinosum and results in a

small growth or wart which is raised above the surface of the skin. Abnormal keratinisation takes place, the cell nuclei are not removed and the granular layer is absent in the wart area. Warts often disappear without treatment but they are contagious and the cosmetician should not touch a wart on a client's skin. Any warts appearing on the hands of a cosmetician should be removed under medical supervision.

There are several types of wart including plane, common and plantar warts. Plane warts are small flesh-coloured flat-topped warts raised above the surface of the skin, often occurring on the hands, knees or face of children. Common warts are usually larger with a much rougher surface and occur on the face or hands of children or young adults. Plantar warts are ingrowing on the soles of the feet and are very painful; they should be treated by a chiropodist.

Herpes simplex (cold sore)

Cold sore (see Fig. 6.3) is a recurring condition due to the presence of a virus in the lower epidermis. The infection is usually contracted in childhood and the virus remains in the skin for a considerable time. The symptoms, however, only appear in times of stress, if a person has a cold, is over-tired or has been over-exposed to the sun or wind. The sore develops as an irritable, itchy patch of vesicles on a red base, followed by crusts which often ooze moisture. There is no specific treatment, though the application of spirit lotion may help. The condition usually clears after a few days. Antiseptic lotions may be applied to prevent secondary bacterial infection. The use of cosmetics in the area should be avoided until the sore heals.

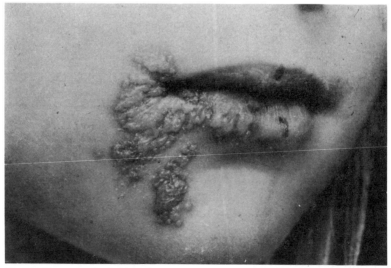

Fig. 6.3 Herpes simplex (cold sore)

Herpes zoster (shingles)

The virus causing this painful complaint is thought to remain dormant in the body following childhood infection by chicken-pox virus. Shingles is most common in the middle-aged and elderly. The onset is marked by itching and erythema of the skin. Vesicles then develop along the pathway of a sensory nerve, sometimes involving those in the skin of the face. The vesicles dry up without rupture, leaving a crust which heals slowly in about two weeks. Pain may, however, persist for several months. In severe cases, pustules may form due to secondary bacterial infection and scarring may occur later. Medical attention is required and no make-up should be applied to the areas involved.

Fungal infections

Fungi which attack the skin, causing various types of ringworm, consist of a series of finely branching threads known as a mycelium. The threads secrete a digestive juice containing a keratin-splitting enzyme. The fungus thus uses keratin for its nutrition and may attack the epidermis, hair or nails but does not invade any living tissue. Any part of the skin, including that of the face, may be affected.

Body ringworm (tinea corporis)

This type of ringworm (see Fig. 6.4) affects the trunk, face or limbs. It is characterised by circular scaly lesions which spread outwards and then

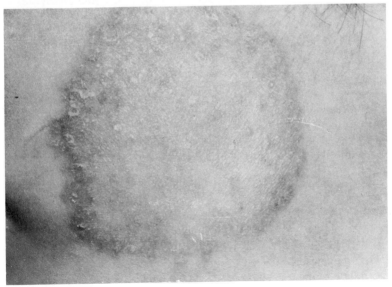

Fig. 6.4 Body ringworm

heal from the centre leaving a ring. Some papules and pustules may
,develop. Medical attention is necessary and no cosmetic service should
be offered if ringworm is suspected. Treatment is by the drug griseofulvin
taken orally.

Disorders affecting the sebaceous glands

Disorders affecting the sebaceous glands may be due to under- or over-
activity of the glands, or to retention of sebum and keratin scales in the
hair follicles with possible bacterial infection.

Asteatosis

The under-activity of the sebaceous glands or asteatosis is rare and is
usually associated with another condition such as hypothyroidism or with
old age. The skin is flaky and dry with a tendency to itching and cracking,
particularly in cold weather. Treatment is by emollient creams.

Seborrhoea

Seborrhoea or excess secretion of sebum in certain areas of the skin is a
common complaint. On the face, the follicle openings in the naso-labial
folds and forehead may become enlarged and blocked by sebum and
keratin scales. The secretion of sebum is controlled by hormones and it is
the change in hormone level at puberty which is responsible for excessive
sebaceous activity, a predisposing factor to the development of acne in
adolescents. Frequent and thorough cleansing using a non-greasy cleanser is required. Any thick creams, pastes or powders which may block the
pores should be avoided.

Comedones (blackheads)

When a plug of dried sebum and keratin scales fills the opening of a hair
follicle, a blackhead or comedo may be formed. The head of the plug is
darkened due to oxidation by the air rather than to dirt. Acne may follow
if the blocked follicle becomes inflamed. If uninfected, blackheads may
be squeezed out but there is a danger of pushing some of the blockage
lower into the follicle with consequent infection and possible scarring.

Acne vulgaris (simple acne)

Acne is a chronic inflammatory disorder due to blockage of follicles with
sebum and keratin, followed by comedones, papules and pustules. Bacteria break down the sebum, forming highly irritant fatty acids which
seep into the surrounding dermis causing inflammation. Red papules
form which may later develop into yellow-headed pustules eventually
discharging pus. Since the follicle opening is blocked, newly produced

sebum cannot escape and the contents of the follicle may be pushed deep into the dermis, forming a cyst. Skin repair after acne often leaves the skin pitted or lumpy and can be very disfiguring. Medical aid is required if the condition persists or if it is at all severe. Acne often starts at puberty and usually clears by the age of 20; it is not thought to be affected by diet. Frequent de-greasing of the area is required and treatment by a 1 per cent solution of cetrimide is useful as an antiseptic. Cosmetics which may block the pores should be avoided.

Steatoma (sebaceous cysts or wens)

Retention of sebum sometimes occurs and collects under the skin as a small nodule called a sebaceous cyst or a wen. The size may vary from that of a pea to a small egg. The cysts occur most frequently in the seborrhoeic areas of the scalp, face and axillae. Some cysts have a small opening and the unpleasant rancid smelling fatty contents can be squeezed out. Cysts with no opening may be removed by incision under local anaesthetic under medical supervision but, as they are considered harmless, they are usually left alone unless very large or inconveniently placed. Normal cosmetic treatment may be given.

Milia (whiteheads)

Milia are small, hard, pearly-white cysts formed of sebum and keratin occurring at the mouth of hair follicles. They have no surface opening as the epidermis covers the cyst. Whiteheads are harmless but often persist for some time, especially around the eyes, on people with dry skin. They may be removed by a doctor or beauty therapist using a sterilised needle.

Rosacea

Rosacea (see Fig. 6.5) is a chronic inflammatory condition affecting the nose, cheeks and forehead, forming a symmetrical butterfly pattern over

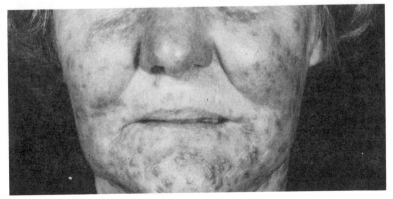

Fig. 6.5 Rosacea

the centre of the face. It is most common in fair-skinned middle-aged women. At first there may be simple blotching of the facial skin and later longer periods of flushing, eventually becoming permanent. The sebaceous glands may be enlarged and some swelling of the nose may occur. Spicy foods, hot tea and coffee, and alcohol tend to cause flushing of the face and should be avoided. Medical attention is advisable. No cosmetic treatment should be given.

Disorders of the sweat glands

Few disorders of the sweat glands will be met with in the salon. The main problem is one of excessive sweating, especially of the feet and axillae, which may lead to embarrassment due to odour and, in the case of the underarm, to wetting of the clothing. If this is the problem of the cosmetician herself and the condition cannot be controlled by the methods suggested below, medical help should be sought.

Hyperidrosis (excessive perspiration)

Excessive perspiration is usually limited to the areas of the hands, feet and axillae where sweat glands are most numerous. It may be a congenital condition but is usually an emotional problem since sweat glands are under nervous control. Frequent bathing, the use of astringents and the liberal use of talcum powder are indicated. Antiperspirants containing astringents such as aluminium chlorhydrate may be used to check underarm perspiration. They are often formulated with deodorants in the form of antiseptics, e.g. hexachlorophene or cetrimide, to prevent the multiplication of bacteria which cause odour by the breakdown of sweat.

Prickly heat (miliaria rubra)

The symptoms of prickly heat are the itching of the skin, the production of small red vesicles and the inflammation of the sweat glands. The complaint may be caused by exposure to excessive heat, usually tropical conditions, or by the closure of the sweat ducts by keratin plugs. It may be treated by frequent bathing and the use of astringents and talcum powder.

Disorders of pigmentation

Pigmented blemishes are often the cause of personal distress and embarrassment but in many cases, especially if the blemish is of normal skin texture and level with the surrounding skin, the area is easily camouflaged by cosmetics. Indeed, moles have sometimes been highlighted as beauty spots.

Freckles (ephelides)

A freckle or ephelis is a small brown macule produced by a group of very active melanocytes in the epidermis. Freckles often first appear on the nose and cheeks of fair-skinned, blonde or red-haired children at about the age of five. Exposure to ultra-violet rays in sunlight causes darkening of the melanin in the freckles, and over-exposure may lead to them extending to form larger brown patches. Freckled skin tends to sunburn easily so avoidance of sunlight, or the use of sun screen creams, is recommended. Freckles tend to fade during the winter months. They may be concealed by cosmetic camouflage.

Lentigines

A lentigo is a congenitally formed area of brown pigmented skin usually larger than a freckle. However, unlike freckles, lentigines do not darken on exposure to sunlight.

Senile lentigines or age spots are similar brown patches which develop on the face and hands of older people. These are increased by sunlight, and sun screen creams may be helpful. Cosmetic camouflage may be used to conceal the blemishes.

Chloasma

Chloasma is an increase of pigmentation occurring during pregnancy or sometimes as a result of taking certain types of contraceptive pills, and is due to the stimulation of melanin production by the female hormone oestrogen. Areas of the face especially round the eyes, the pubic area and the nipples are most usually affected. Brown patches on the face may be treated by cosmetic camouflage. The excess colour usually disappears gradually when the pregnancy ends or the use of contraceptives is discontinued.

Vitiligo (leucoderma)

Vitiligo (see Fig. 6.6) is caused by the complete absence of colour in usually small but definite areas of the skin due to melanocyte destruction. The condition is more obvious in darker skins. The skin is of normal texture and the condition can be concealed by cosmetic camouflage. For white-skinned people, sun tanning should be avoided since this makes the white patches more obvious by increasing the contrast.

Albinism

Albinism is a congenital defect in which melanocytes are present but are unable to produce melanin. Pigment is absent throughout the body so that albinos have fair skin, blonde hair and no colour in the iris of the eyes.

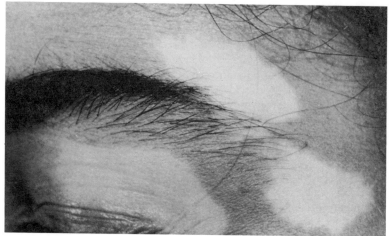

Fig. 6.6 Vitiligo on black skin

Haemangioma

These are vascular lesions due to areas of permanently dilated capillaries. The lesions include port wine stains, strawberry marks and spider naevi.

Port wine stain (capillary naevus or naevus flammeus)
This is a flat, red or purple, usually quite large, area of permanently dilated capillaries, often covering one side of the face (see Fig. 6.7). It is usually present at birth and persists throughout life. The blemish may be concealed by cosmetic camouflage. Dermatological treatment may be possible using laser beam therapy.

Strawberry mark (cavernous naevus or naevus vasculosus)
A strawberry mark is a small bright red area of capillaries which appears on the skin at birth or within a few weeks of birth. It is soft and raised, often with several lobes, and is due to the multiplication of capillaries in the dermis. The mark may slightly increase in size over the first few years, but most disappear by the age of five and the remainder by the age of ten leaving normal skin. No treatment is usually necessary.

Spider telangiectases (spider naevi)
These consist of dilated capillaries radiating like a spider's legs from a central point. Sometimes known as oestrogen spiders, they often increase when oestrogen levels rise as in liver diseases or in pregnancy. They may be removed by cauterising the central point. Green corrective cream is used in cosmetic camouflage.

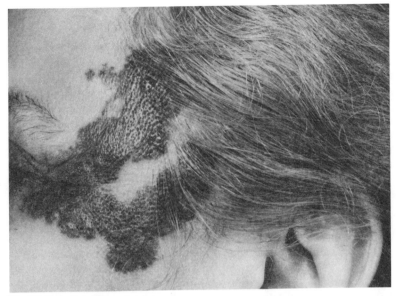

Fig. 6.7 Port wine stain

Broken capillaries (telangiectases)

Sometimes also called broken veins, these small lesions are permanently dilated capillaries rather than being broken. They form on dry, sensitive or neglected skin, and the numbers usually increase with age. Extremes of treatment and temperature should be avoided. They may be camouflaged by green corrective cream.

Moles (melanocytic naevi or melanoma)

Moles consist of accumulations of cells related to melanocytes which lie deep in the dermis. The mole may be present at birth, or may develop later by growth of cells which were already in the skin at birth. Moles are slightly raised above the surface of the skin forming flat-topped soft swellings which may be flesh-coloured or pigmented brown or black. Any hair growing from a mole should not be plucked but should be cut using sterilised scissors. Moles may be surgically removed if they are awkwardly placed but generally speaking they should not be interfered with as they occasionally become cancerous. If a pigmented area appears around a mole or there is any change in size, medical advice should be sought. Normal cosmetic treatment may be given.

Disorders involving abnormal growth

Psoriasis

A tendency to psoriasis is inherited and it usually affects several members of the same family. The condition occurs as oval or round patches of silvery scales which are thicker and larger than normal epidermal scales. The underlying skin is red due to an increase in size and number of dermal capillaries in the area. There are small bleeding points if the scales are removed, but no weeping and no vesicles develop. Some itching may occur. Any area of the skin may be affected but the face, scalp, knees and elbows are common sites. There may be thimble-pitting of the finger nails.

Psoriasis is due to faulty keratinisation. The cell nuclei are still present in the scales and there is an increased rate of cell division in the basal layer. The patches sometimes clear, especially in summer due to the action of ultra-violet rays in sunlight, but they tend to recur in times of stress, indicating some nervous origin of the disease. Medical advice is indicated. Traditional treatment was the removal of the scales by use of coal tar and salicylic acid ointment. More recently, irradiation with ultra-violet rays and application of vitamin A have been used, and also treatment with the steriod triamcinolone. No infection is involved so normal cosmetic treatment may be carried out.

Hypertrichosis and hirsutism

If terminal hair grows in regions normally bearing only vellus type hair, the condition is known as *hypertrichosis*. This may be due to hormone imbalance or an inherited tendency, but often the cause is unknown. The growth of facial hair in a woman often increases due to hormonal changes at the menopause or may be a side effect of taking certain drugs. The growth of hair in typically male sites by a female is known as *hirsutism*.

If hair growth is slight, bleaching is effective in making dark hairs less noticeable and also tends to weaken hairs often causing breakage. Chemical depilatories should be used on the face with caution since the skin in that area is sensitive. Manufacturers' instructions regarding use should be followed. Waxing is often used as an alternative or single hairs may be plucked. More permanent methods of removal by diathermy (electrolysis) should be carried out by a qualified and experienced person as there is considerable danger of scarring.

Skin tags

These often appear on the neck area in the elderly. They are small growths of fibrous tissue which stand away from the skin. Sometimes they are pigmented black or brown which makes them more obvious. They may be removed by a doctor if they prove to be a nuisance.

Allergies

An allergy is an abnormal reaction or hypersensitivity of the body tissue of an individual to a substance which does not affect the majority of people. The substance causing the reaction is called an *allergen*. Some allergens may be substances taken internally as in drugs, e.g. penicillin, or foods such as strawberries or eggs. They may also be inhaled, e.g. pollen which gives rise to hay fever, and house mites or cat hairs which cause sneezing and watering of the eyes in some people. Medical advice is often required to determine the nature of the allergy.

The allergies of most concern to cosmeticians are those caused by substances on external contact with the skin. These external allergens give rise to *contact eczema* or *contact dermatitis*. Strictly speaking, dermatitis refers to the inflammation of the skin, while eczema refers to tissue reactions involving erythema, weeping, blisters, swelling and scaling of the skin, but the two terms are often used interchangeably.

External chemical irritants are called *primary irritants* if they cause inflammation at the first contact, and the irritation is confined to the area of contact. Caustic liquids such as strong acids and alkalis are primary irritants. Some detergents will also cause dermatitis in all people if applied in sufficient concentration and for sufficient time.

A chemical may be a *secondary irritant* or *sensitiser* if it causes inflammation only in particular people who have become allergic to the substance through previous contact. In this case the reaction is not confined to the area of contact but may affect any area. On first exposure the sensitiser produces no visible sign of irritation but causes the formation of anti-bodies in the blood, which then react against the substance on any subsequent application. The body thus becomes allergic to the substance and it must then never be applied to the skin again, even in very low concentrations. Reaction to the allergen may involve slight erythema, or may result in the formation of vesicles with weeping and swelling of the tissues, in which case medical advice is necessary.

Substances used in the manufacture of cosmetics which are liable to cause dermatitis include lanolin, paratoluenediamine used in eyelash dyes, formaldehyde resins used in nail enamels, and the essential oils of bergamot, lavender and cedarwood used in perfumes. Other substances which often become sensitisers include some drugs, e.g. penicillin, antihistamine creams used to treat insect bites, metals such as traces of nickel and chromium which often occur in jewellery, and some plants, e.g. primulas.

Hypo-allergenic cosmetics are available, in which known allergens such as lanolin, formaldehyde resins and eosin (a lipstick dye) are avoided. It is, however, impossible to prepare non-allergenic products since different people are susceptible to different substances. Hypo-allergenic products usually contain no preservatives or perfumes and the amount of colour is often reduced.

Urticaria (hives)

Urticaria is a short-lived reaction of the skin to an allergen or to firm stroking in which weals are formed. There is some swelling of the dermis, the skin is itchy, and a red area surrounds a raised white portion of skin. The rash appears quickly and usually disappears without trace within a day or two.

Questions

1. What is meant by (a) an allergen and (b) a hypo-allergenic cosmetic? Give four examples of substances used in cosmetics which often cause allergic reaction.
2. Name four diseases or conditions which (a) are contra-indicative of cosmetic treatment and (b) may be treated by cosmetic camouflage.
3. What features would distinguish:
    (a) a boil from a carbuncle;
    (b) freckles from lentigines;
    (c) a wart from a mole;
    (d) a port wine stain from a strawberry mark?
4. What advice would you give to a client who:
    (a) complained of brown patches appearing on her face during pregnancy;
    (b) developed a series of broken capillaries;
    (c) was concerned about the growth of facial hair around her mouth?
5. Which disorders of the skin are associated with ageing? Suggest the treatment and advice which should be offered in each case.

Chapter 7

Cleansing, toning and moisturising

Preparation of the skin by cleansing, toning and moisturising is essential before the re-application of make-up. Equipment should be already sterilised and the trolley set out before the client arrives. Preparation of the client for treatment and analysis of the facial skin must be carried out before cleansing begins.

Preparation of the equipment

The cosmetician's hands must be scrupulously clean before commencing the preparation.

The required equipment and materials are listed below.

Trolley or tray
Spatulas (wooden or plastic)
Cotton wool pads (damp)
Tissues
Selection of cleansers for different skin types
Selection of toners for different skin types
Selection of moisturisers
Sterilising fluid (for insertion of spatulas)
Headband
Gown, cape or towels
Record card

The trolley or tray should have been cleaned using a disinfectant. On removal from the ultra-violet cabinet, spatulas should be placed in sterilising fluid or laid on a clean tissue. Bottles and pots should be free from drips, and kept clean and tidy throughout the treatment. Before showing in the client, the trolley must be checked to ensure that all the equipment is present and adequate amounts of materials have been prepared in order to avoid leaving the client once treatment has started.

Preparation of the client (see Fig. 7.1)

Ideally the client should be in a reclining position, either on a chair which will tilt or on a couch. A safe and secure position is essential so that the client feels relaxed at all times. In particular, the head and shoulders should be well supported. The cosmetician needs clear access to both the head and neck, with the client at a suitable height in order to avoid undue stress or fatigue to the cosmetician during treatment. If it is necessary for the client to remove her shoes to enable her to recline fully, a towel may be wrapped round the feet and legs for added comfort.

At this stage the client should be requested to remove ear-rings, necklaces etc. and these must be kept in a place of safety. A clean headband is necessary round the hairline to ensure that all the client's hair is kept well away from the face, and a protective cover secured across the front of the client to avoid the possible soiling of clothing.

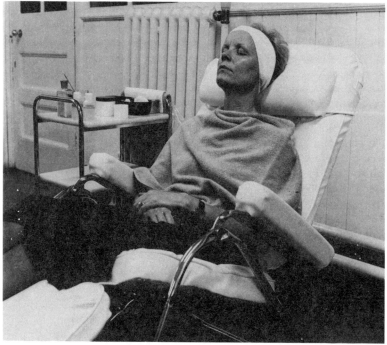

Fig. 7.1 Preparation of client for cleansing

Skin analysis

Before the commencement of any make-up procedure, the skin must be analysed in order to select the preparations appropriate to the particular client. Certain details should be noted before making the correct selection of materials. These are as follows:

1. Is the skin dry? (The signs are flaking, lack of moisture and the presence of milia.)
2. Is the skin greasy? (The signs are shiny skin, open pores, blackheads and possibly a sallow appearance.)

3. Are there other skin blemishes, such as broken capillaries? (Broken capillaries would usually be seen around the cheeks.)
4. Does the client have acne or any other skin problem?
5. The skin's general condition should be noted. Is it soft and smooth or harsh and rough?
6. Has the client ever experienced an allergic reaction to any cosmetic preparation?

On completion of the analysis, the results should be recorded on a skin analysis chart (see Fig. 7.2). The cosmetician will then be able to select the following:

(a) An appropriate cleaner.
(b) The correct toning lotion or bracer.
(c) The correct moisturiser.
(d) The type of mask required.

Skin analysis chart

Name of client............   Date.............................

Skin   Skin
characteristics .... treatment....................
Skin type .... Type of
Colour....................... cleanser ....
Texture...................... Type of toner ....
Abnormalities .... Type of
.... moisturiser.................
                              Type of mask............

Allergies ....
Muscle tone ....

Fig. 7.2 Skin analysis chart

If the client is wearing make-up, skin analysis is made more difficult since the skin itself is not so easily seen. In this case the cosmetician would need to ask the client to give information about her skin, and then make an analysis from the information given. After the first cleanse the skin would obviously be visible, and a more detailed analysis could then be made if necessary.

Cleansing the skin

The purpose of cleansing is to remove the following from the skin's surface:

(a) Stale make-up (often oil-based).
(b) Excess sebum which may be solidified in the openings of the hair follicles, causing enlarged pores.
(c) Water-soluble solids left on the skin after the evaporation of perspiration.
(d) Grime and dust.
(e) Skin debris, i.e. loose dead scales of keratin.

Thus the cleansing agent must be capable of removing both oil-soluble and water-soluble substances. Cleansing is usually achieved by the use of soap and water, or by emulsions in the form of cleansing creams or lotions.

Cleansing preparations

1. Soap and water
Soap and water is an effective cleanser for normal skins. Soap acts as an emulsifying agent and so helps to remove grease from the skin by emulsifying it. Water dissolves any water-soluble substances on the skin. Insoluble particles of dirt and skin cells are usually removed mechanically during the cleansing process. The soap should be superfatted (that is, it should have added vegetable oils to reduce its alkalinity) and should be rinsed away using soft water since hard water is considered to be drying to the skin. Finally, the skin should be patted dry with a towel rather than rubbed. For dry and sensitive skins, cleansing creams are a more effective alternative to soap and water. Cleansing creams are also essential for removing very oily make-up from the area around the eyes.

2. Cleansing creams and lotions (emulsions)
The effectiveness of cleansing creams can be demonstrated by the fact that if they are used after washing the face with soap and water, further cleansing takes place. Creams are especially efficient in removing hardened sebum from the hair follicles.

Cleansing creams may be formulated as either oil-in-water or water-in-oil emulsions, whereas lotions are normally oil-in-water emulsions only. Both act on the skin in the same way. The oil of the emulsion dissolves grease (sebum and oily make-up) and the water in the emulsion dissolves any water-soluble substances. Insoluble particles of dirt and flakes of keratin are dislodged mechanically and removed with the emulsion when it is wiped off the face.

The main difference between creams and lotions is in the proportion of oils they contain. Creams contain 40–50 per cent oil and lotions only 10–25 per cent. Thus creams are usually preferred for cleansing dry skins and lotions for greasy skins. Lotions being more liquid are easier to apply. Creams should spread evenly over the skin without drag, and should be easily removed with a tissue or cotton wool pad leaving the skin smooth but non-greasy. Since these preparations have a short contact time with the skin, they have little moisturising effect or skin penetration.

Traditional cleansing creams were called *cold creams* since the evaporation of moisture from the emulsion caused cooling of the skin.

The composition of cleansing creams and lotions is shown in Table 7.1.

Table 7.1 Composition of cleansing creams and lotions

Types of cleanser	Oil phase	Use
O/W cold cream	40–60% almond oil	For dry skin
O/W cleansing cream	40–60% oils (mineral oil with some vegetable oil)	For dry skin
W/O cleansing cream	40–60% oils and waxes (mineral oil, lanolin, vegetable oil, ozokerite)	For dry skin
Hypo-allergenic cream	As W/O cleansing cream without lanolin	For sensitive skin
O/W cleansing lotion	10–25% mineral oil	For greasy skin

3. Other cleansers

(a) *Liquefying creams* containing no water are useful for the removal of water-proof eye make-up such as non-aqueous eye shadow, since they remove only greasy products. The creams contain mineral oils, petroleum jelly and waxes such as spermaceti and ozokerite. The cream is solid in the jar but liquefies on contact with the skin.

(b) *Non-greasy preparations* contain only triethanolamine lauryl sulphate (a soapless detergent) and water, or sometimes sulphonated oils and water. These are most useful for very greasy skins.

The cleansing procedure

Cleansing takes place in two stages. A superficial cleanse removes surface grease and dirt. This is followed by a deep cleanse to ensure that all traces of make-up, dirt and grease are removed from the face, leaving it clean and grease-free in preparation for further treatment.

The superficial cleanse (see Fig. 7.3)

1. Wash your hands thoroughly.
2. Select the correct cleanser according to the client's skin type.

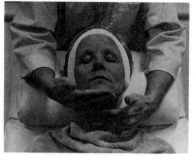

(a) Use effleurage (stroking) movements from the base of the neck up to the tip of the chin, one hand following the other.

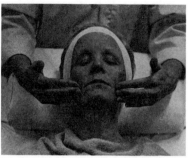

(b) Use rotary movements over the cheek area, both hands working simultaneously.

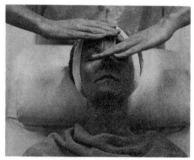

(c) Gently glide the hands up from the cheeks around the outside of the eyes to the centre of the forehead. Then, using one hand after the other, carry out effleurage movements down the nose.

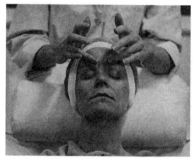

(d) Using the ring finger of each hand, trace a circle around the outer eye, working outwards and back towards the nose.

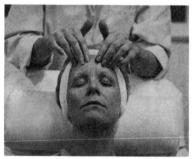

(e) Use the fingers of each hand to carry out small circular movements over the forehead, working from one side to the other.

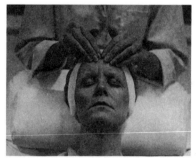

(f) To finish, gently glide the hands down the outside of the eyes to the chin. Then make a circular movement back up to the cheeks and a further circular movement up to the forehead. Apply slight pressure to the centre forehead, pause and then lift the hands away.

Fig. 7.3 Superficial cleanse

3. With a sterilised spatula remove sufficient cream from the jar to complete the treatment and place it on the back of your non-working hand. Alternatively, if using a lotion, pour the cleanser directly into the palm of your hand.
4. Apply the cleanser to the neck and face (avoiding the eyes and lips) using an upwards stroking movement with the pads of the fingers. Use sufficient cream to avoid dragging the skin. The sequence of movements used during the superficial cleanse are shown in Fig. 7.3.
5. Remove the cleanser using damp cotton wool pads or tissues, again employing upward movements.
6. Apply cleanser to the eyes and lips and again remove with damp cotton wool or tissues (see Fig. 7.4 (a) and (b)). If mascara is being removed, a damp cotton wool pad should be placed under the eye to prevent it from staining the skin. A protected orange stick may be used to remove any stubborn areas of mascara. Extreme care should be taken when working round the eyes since the skin of this area is thin and easily damaged. The eyes and lips may either be cleansed at the beginning or at the end of the treatment, but should always be treated separately from the remainder of the face.

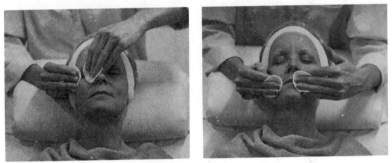

Fig. 7.4 (a) Cleansing the eyes, (b) Cleansing the lips

The deep cleanse

A more intricate massage is carried out during the deep cleanse. There are numerous methods of massage but, irrespective of the method used, the basic principles and the relevant safety precautions should be observed. The massage should not be too deep. It should aim to stimulate the blood supply and this, in turn, will help to increase the secretion of sweat and sebum through the pores of the skin so removing waste products. The superficial layer of the stratum corneum is also removed by massage, leaving a smoother surface. The massage movements should always be upwards and outwards to avoid stretching the skin. A suitable sequence of massage movements for a deep cleanse is shown in Fig. 7.5.

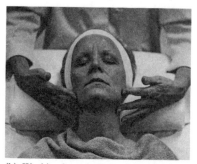

(a) Working from the base óf the neck, use effleurage (stroking) movements up to the chin. Draw the hands outwards along the jawline to the ears. Then gently drop down to the base of the neck and repeat the procedure about 6 times.

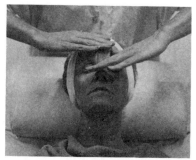

(b) Working from the base of the ears along the jawline, project the index finger along the bottom of the jawline, lift up on to the chin and glide back to the ears, working with one hand first followed by the other.

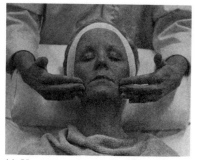

(c) Use rotary movements over the cheek area, both hands working simultaneously.

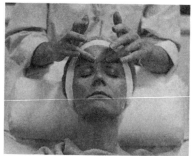

(d) Gently glide the hands up from the cheeks around the outside of the eyes to the centre forehead. Then, using one hand after the other, carry out effleurage movements down the nose.

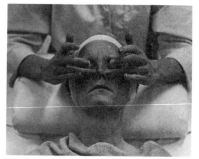

(e) Bring the fingers of each hand down the sides of the nose so that both fingers meet at the centre under the nose. Then, using a circular movement, take the fingers back up the sides of the nose and repeat this about 6 times.

(f) Gently glide the ring fingers up the sides of the nose to the centre of the forehead. Trace a circle around the outer eye, working outward then back towards the nose again. Repeat 6 times.

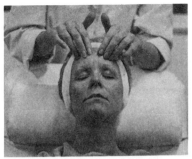

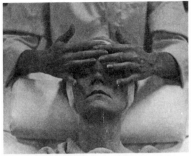

(g) Use the fingers of each hand to carry out small circular movements over the forehead, working from one side to the other.

(h) Using the fingers of both hands, carry out a scissor action across the forehead from one side to the other.

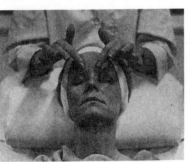

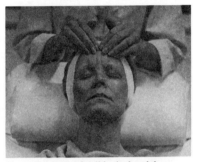

(i) Place the ring finger of each hand at the centre forehead. Working outwards, trace a line around the outer eye, bringing the fingers back to the centre forehead. Then, using the index finger followed by the middle finger and then the ring finger, carry out tapotement (tapping movements) gently over the brow bone. Repeat 6 times.

(j) To finish, gently glide the hand down the outside of the eyes, down to the chin, make a circular movement back up to the cheeks then a further circular movement up to the forehead. Apply slight pressure to the centre forehead, pause and then lift the hands away.

Fig. 7.5 Deep cleanse

Toning

On completion of the deep cleanse, the cream is removed using damp cotton wool with an upwards movement and the skin is then toned to ensure that no traces remain. The toner will also produce a cooling sensation, refreshing the skin and closing the pores.

There are three types of toner.

1. Astringent lotions

These are the strongest toners and are used on greasy skins which show no signs of sensitivity, or on young spotty skins. Astringents are substances which cause contraction of the skin tissues and so help to close the pores. Witch hazel (obtained from the leaves and twigs of a plant), menthol (obtained from oil of peppermint) and aluminium chlorhydrate are suitable astringents for use in these lotions. The main astringent, however, is always alcohol (ethanol) and astringent lotions may contain up to 40 per cent of it. Since it is a volatile liquid, alcohol evaporates rapidly at skin temperature. The heat (known as latent heat) required to change the liquid alcohol to its gaseous state during evaporation is taken from the skin itself and so the skin is cooled. The antiseptic properties of alcohol make it suitable for use on spotty skins, but it is drying and may also cause irritation or stinging if applied to sensitive skins. A lotion containing more than 20 per cent alcohol is unsuitable for use on dry or sensitive skin.

Other ingredients in astringent lotions are antiseptics such as hexa-chlorophene, perfumes such as orange flower water or rose water, and emollients such as glycerol.

2. Skin tonics

Slightly milder toners are known as skin tonics. These contain 10–15 per cent alcohol together with small quantities of astringents such as witch hazel. Skin tonics are used on normal skin.

3. Skin bracers or fresheners

The mildest toners, known as skin bracers or fresheners, contain no alcohol. These simple toners consist entirely of purified water, rose water or orange flower water and have only a slightly astringent effect. They cool the skin by evaporation. Fresheners are suitable for use on normal young unblemished skin, on delicate dehydrated mature skin, and on black skin which tends to be sensitive.

Application of toners

There are two alternative methods of application.

1. Using cotton wool pads

(a) Select the appropriate toner according to the client's skin type.
(b) Apply sufficient toner to two damp cotton wool pads. Then, holding one pad in each hand, gently pat the toner over the face and neck.
(c) With upward stroking movements, gently wipe the face and neck with the pads, ensuring that all traces of the cleanser are removed.

2. Using a tonic gauze

The gauze is cut to the face shape as shown in Fig. 7.6 and soaked in the appropriate toner according to the client's skin type before application to the face. The gauze may be left in position for up to 5 minutes. Adaptation is necessary for use on a combination type skin. In this case, the face-shaped gauze should be cut to fit the central oily T-panel and this part soaked in tonic. The remainder of the gauze should then be soaked with a mild bracer and fitted into position around the T-panel.

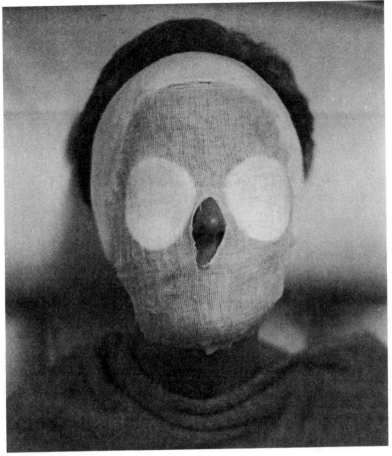

Fig. 7.6 Tonic gauze

Moisturising

Moisturisers are used after toning and before the application of foundation make-up. The moisturising cream or lotion thus acts as a barrier between the skin and the make-up. It eases the application of cosmetics by providing a smooth surface and also facilitates their eventual removal. If no make-up is to be worn, the moisturiser protects the skin from the damaging effect of the wind and sun, and from the drying effect of low humidity in centrally heated rooms. The main purpose of a moisturiser is to keep the skin soft, smooth and supple by maintaining the moisture level of the stratum corneum.

The moisturising effect of these creams and lotions is achieved by:
1. The use of an *oil-in-water emulsion* with a high percentage of water

(up to 70 per cent in creams and 90 per cent in lotions). The water phase has the greater contact with the skin and allows some absorption of water by the stratum corneum.

2. The addition of *a humectant* such as glycerol to attract moisture into the cream from the surrounding air. (The humectant also prevents the cream from drying out in the jar before use.)

3. The *emollient* but non-greasy film left on the skin surface after the evaporation of the water phase. This helps to prevent loss of moisture from the skin and encourages the build-up of moisture from the dermis. The bulk of the oil phase consists of stearic acid though a little mineral oil and lanolin may be included. Stearic acid is a white waxy substance with a melting point above skin temperature, so that tiny waxy crystals are left on the skin. These form the matt non-greasy (and therefore non-shiny) film which is so essential in a day cream. The oily layer also cements down any loose scales of keratin, giving the skin a smoother surface.

Application of moisturisers

Creams containing 15–30 per cent of oil phase are suitable for dry skins and lotions with 10–15 per cent oil for greasy skins. Hypo-allergenic creams and lotions without lanolin are also available. Moisturisers are best applied to a slightly damp skin. This moisture will mix freely with the water phase of the emulsion and aid the absorption of moisture by the horny layer.

The moisturiser is applied by dotting the cream from the back of the non-working hand on to the client's face, then blending in gently with the pads of the fingers. If a moisturising lotion is used, this is poured into the palm and applied in the same way as the cream.

Night creams

The cosmetician may be asked to give advice about the use of night creams. These used to be known as skin foods or nourishing creams and are now sometimes referred to as skin conditioning creams. This type of cream is left on the skin overnight. It helps to repair damage caused by exposure to the wind and sun, and to relieve dryness and roughness. The creams should be easy to apply, but should not be rubbed in too well nor be easily wiped off by the bedclothes. The occlusive oily film should not be absorbed too quickly, so allowing a long contact time on the skin. This enables the emollient properties of the cream to have maximum effect, by delaying loss of moisture from the surface of the epidermis and allowing time for water to build up from the tissues below.

Night creams consist of soft solid or thick liquid cream emulsions with a high oil content. Since they are used only overnight, the shiny appearance of a greasy skin is not important, and they are usually formulated as water-in-oil emulsions. They may contain up to 80 per cent oil if intended for dry skin or only 45 per cent for greasy skin. Mineral oil, vegetable oil and petroleum jelly may be used, often thickened with paraffin wax or ozokerite. Some lanolin may also be included. Night creams may contain added vitamins, or hormones such as oestrogen (a female sex hormone), but the usefulness of these is questionable. Oestrogens are thought to rejuvenate senile skin by restoring the water-holding capacity of ageing skin, but their over-use may have undesirable side effects.

Questions

1. Explain why:
   (a) glycerol is often used as an ingredient of moisturising creams;
   (b) alcohol cools the skin;
   (c) night creams are usually water-in-oil emulsions;
   (d) cleansers have little moisturising effect.
2. What is meant by an astringent? Give two examples of astringent substances. For which types of skin are astringent lotions (a) suitable and (b) unsuitable?
3. Why is the regular use of a moisturiser important?
4. What is the purpose of a cleanser?
   What type of cleanser is most suitable for a client with (a) a very greasy skin and (b) a dry skin?
5. What preparations are necessary to ensure the comfort of both the client and cosmetician during the cleansing and toning of the skin?

Chapter 8

Face masks and packs

The terms 'face mask' and 'face pack' are usually considered to have the same meaning. However, strictly speaking, *a mask* refers to an absorbent piece of material, such as cotton, which is cut to the shape of the face with openings for the eyes, nose and mouth. The mask may be applied to the face as a single piece of material soaked in the active ingredient, e.g. an oil mask, or as double material with the active ingredient between the two layers, e.g. a fruit mask. *Peel-off masks* are also possible in which gels or waxes are painted on the skin and the mask is peeled off in one piece after setting. *A pack* is applied directly to the face in the form of a paste, e.g. a clay pack, or a cream, e.g. a yeast pack, and is not removable in one piece.

Numerous face masks and packs are available to the cosmetician and the choice will depend mainly on the suitability to skin type. They are available in many forms and, depending on the ingredients, can be used to reduce skin irritation or to soothe, moisturise, soften, de-grease, bleach, cleanse, refresh, stimulate or tighten the skin. Heat may be required when using certain preparations.

Preparation of the client

Prior to the application of a face mask or pack, the client should be prepared as for the cleansing process, and the face cleansed to remove all make-up and oils as previously described in Chapter 7. Careful diagnosis of the skin type is essential in order to select the most beneficial pack or mask. The cosmetician should stay with the client throughout treatment so that the preparation may be removed immediately if any discomfort is felt.

Contra-indications to treatment

No pack or mask should be applied:
1. if infection is present, e.g. cold sores or impetigo;
2. where there are cuts or wounds;
3. if the skin is known to be over-sensitive.

Types of masks and packs

Basically there are four types of masks and packs. These may be classified according to their ingredients, and also into setting types (which are
allowed to dry out or solidify on the skin) and non-setting types, as
shown below.
1. *Natural* (non-setting) packs/masks.
2. *Clay based* (setting) packs.
3. *Peel-off masks* (setting) (a) gels, (b) latex, (c) wax.
4. *Warm oil masks* (non-setting).
Proprietary or commercially prepared packs and masks may be either
clay based or of the peel-off variety. As they come ready for use, preparation time is minimal, making them ideal for salon treatments. They are
usually available for all skin types. The manufacturer's instructions regarding use must be strictly followed. The package should include a list
of ingredients, and if this is not available the product should be treated
with care, as any particular client may experience allergic reaction to
some ingredient.

Natural face packs and masks

As the heading implies, these are made from completely natural substances, e.g. fruit and vegetables. They must be prepared immediately
before use as they deteriorate quickly on keeping. Cotton wool eye pads,
moistened with purified water or orange flower water, should be applied
during treatment to relax and refresh the eyes.

Avocado packs
Avocado is an oily fruit and is therefore suitable for dry skin. The fruit is
prepared by mashing it to a pulp, then mixing it to a thin cream by the
addition of egg yolk; a little glycerol may also be added. The mixture
should be applied directly to the face with a brush, left for 15–20 minutes,
then removed with a moist sponge. Blotting the face with damp cotton
wool will remove any remaining traces.

Oatmeal packs
Oatmeal may be mixed to a paste with rose water and applied to the skin
with a brush. It has an abrasive action and is often used as a cleansing
pack on normal or greasy skins. It will improve the skin's texture and
should be left on for 15 minutes.

   Oatmeal may also be mixed to a paste with honey and applied to the
skin in the same way. This again will cleanse the skin and have a softening effect. Oatmeal packs should be removed with tepid water on cotton
wool pads.

Cucumber masks
After removing the rind, the cucumber is sliced thinly. The slices may
then be either applied directly to the face or, alternatively, placed be-

tween two pieces of fine gauze before application. The gauze must previously have been cut to the shape of the face with holes made for the eyes, nose and mouth. The mask is left for 20 minutes before removal. Slices of cucumber may be used as eye pads. The cucumber acts as an astringent and cools the skin. The mask is suitable for normal and greasy skins.

Crushed strawberries may be used in the same way.

Egg packs

For dry skins the egg yolk only is used. It may be whisked together with honey before application. The pack is left for 20 minutes and then removed with cotton wool pads and water.

The white of an egg may be whipped until quite stiff before application to the skin. This is ideal for greasy skins and will also have a tightening effect. If the face is exceedingly oily, a few drops of lemon juice may be added to the egg white. The pack is left for 20 minutes or until dry, and then removed with warm water and cotton wool pads.

Fruit masks and packs

It is possible to create many natural fruit face masks and packs by using in particular the citrus fruits and also bananas, apples etc. They may be crushed and used between gauze or applied directly to the skin. Alternatively, they may be mixed with egg white to form a cream and applied directly to the face. They are normally left for 15–20 minutes and then removed by warm water and cotton wool pads. If it is noticed that the client's skin becomes sensitive to any mask or pack, it should be removed immediately.

Yeast packs

Brewers' yeast is used and is mixed to a smooth paste with witch hazel for greasy skin or with rose water for dry skin. The mixture should be of a thickish consistency otherwise it will run off the face. It should be applied with a face mask brush, avoiding the eyes and mouth. After leaving for 15–20 minutes it may be removed with tepid water and cotton wool pads. Yeast both cleanses and softens the skin.

Clay-based packs

Clay packs are essentially cleansing packs since the clay absorbs excess sebum and sweat as well as aiding desquamation. Dead cells from the superficial layer of the stratum corneum and particles of dirt become embedded in the clay and are removed with it at the end of the treatment. The packs are prepared by mixing clays and other powdered ingredients with liquids such as purified water or witch hazel, according to the type of skin to be treated. The mixture can be adjusted to suit any particular type of skin. The packs are normally left on until they have completely dried out.

The powdered ingredients include the following substances.

(a) *Kaolin* or china clay (a hydrous aluminium silicate)
Kaolin is a white to pale cream slightly abrasive powder and is therefore useful for cleansing acnefied skin. It is particularly effective in bringing blind acne spots to a head and removing comedones. For this purpose, on greasy skins the kaolin is mixed with fuller's earth and witch hazel, for normal skins kaolin is mixed with purified water, and for dry skins with calamine and rose water.

(b) *Fuller's earth* (another form of hydrous aluminium silicate)
This clay is a grey powder with a stronger action than kaolin and sometimes causes reddening of the skin. It has a deep cleansing action with good absorbency, so is particularly useful on greasy skin when mixed with witch hazel. For normal skin it could be mixed with rose water or purified water. It can also be mixed with kaolin, magnesium carbonate or sulphur according to the remedial effect required.

(c) *Bentonite* (also a form of hydrous aluminium silicate)
Bentonite is a grey-white clay obtained from volcanic ash. It swells in water and has good absorbency properties; it is often used in commercially prepared packs. Titinium dioxide or zinc oxide is sometimes added to the pack to improve the appearance by making it whiter.

(d) *Light magnesium carbonate*
This is a mildly astringent white powder suitable for skin with open pores. It has a toning effect and softens and refines the skin. Magnesium carbonate is usually added to one of the clays mentioned above to give bulk, but may be used alone as the basis of a pack for normal or dry skin when it should be mixed with either rose water or purified water.

(e) *Sulphur*
Sulphur is available in the form of a fine yellow powder. It is rarely used as a pack on its own, but may be added in small quantities to fuller's earth for use on extremely greasy skin. On acnefied skin or skin with blackheads, it may be applied to the actual blemishes themselves before application of a fuller's earth pack. Packs containing sulphur are usually mixed with witch hazel.

(f) *Calamine*
Calamine is a pale pink powder containing zinc carbonate which is soothing to inflamed skin. It may therefore be added to packs intended for sensitive or delicate skin and may be mixed with magnesium carbonate or kaolin depending on the desired effect. Calamine may also be used on its own for dry sensitive skin, and is usually mixed with rose water or purified water. On extremely dry skin it may be mixed with a vegetable oil such as almond oil, in which case the pack will not dry out completely.

The liquids used to mix clay-based packs include the following:

(a)*Witch hazel*
Witch hazel is an astringent liquid and is drying to the skin. It is used on greasy skin but never on dry or sensitive skin. If a slight reaction is shown to witch hazel, it may be diluted with rose water or purified water.

(b) *Rose water and orange flower water*
These perfumed waters are mildly toning and may be used to mix packs intended for use on dry or sensitive skin.

(c) *Soft or purified water*
These are suitable for mixing packs for normal skin. Hard water is not used as the salts it contains are considered to be drying to the skin.

(d) *Vegetable oils*
Oils, such as almond oil and sulphonated castor oil, may be used to mix calamine packs for use on exceedingly dry skin. Small quantities of oils may also be added to clay packs to keep the clay more flexible, so aiding removal and having a moisturising effect on dry skin.

(e) *Glycerol*
Glycerol, a humectant, may be added to packs intended for dry or de-hydrated skin. The humectant helps to retain water in the pack itself and prevents it from drying out completely.

(f) *Hydrogen peroxide*
Dilute solutions of hydrogen peroxide (5 volume) may be used to give the pack a lightening or slight bleaching effect for use on black skin. Clay packs, however, are not usually popular with dark-skinned people since they tend to leave white streaks on the skin.

Preparation of clay packs
A careful appraisal of the skin should always be made prior to giving a face pack. By experience, the cosmetician should be able to judge the quantities and mixture required for a client, taking into account the area to be covered and the effect required. A summary of suitable packs according to skin types is shown in Table 8.1.

The required solid ingredients should be placed in a bowl and mixed to a smooth paste by gradually adding the chosen liquid so that no irritant particles remain. The paste must not be too thin or it will tend to run off the face. Nor must it be too thick, making it difficult to apply and inhibit-ing the drying time.

Application and removal of clay packs
1. Warn the client that the pack may feel cold when first applied.
2. Using a mask brush, quickly apply a thin film of paste evenly over the face, starting at the chin and working upwards.

Table 8.1 Suggestions for clay packs

Skin type	Powdered ingredients	Liquid ingredients
Normal skin	Calamine or fuller's earth	Purified water
Dry skin	Calamine	Rose water
Greasy skin	Fuller's earth	Witch hazel
Combination skin	Greasy area fuller's earth	Witch hazel
	Dry area calamine	Rose water
Sensitive skin	Calamine	Rose water
Acnefied skin	Kaolin and fuller's earth	Witch hazel
Greasy skin with open pores	Magnesium carbonate and fuller's earth	Witch hazel
Dry skin with open pores	Magnesium carbonate and calamine	Rose water

3. Extreme care should be taken to avoid contact with the eyes, and the paste should be kept away from the mouth and nostrils.
4. If two types of clay are being used on a combination skin, the one requiring the longer treatment time should be applied first so that the two can be removed together.
5. The eyes may be covered with cotton wool pads soaked in orange flower water.
6. The client should experience a slight tightening of the skin as the pack shrinks a little on drying.
7. When the pack has dried out sufficiently, it should be removed gently with warm dampened towels. Any residual matter may be cleaned away by use of a sponge and warm water.
8. The treatment should be followed by the application of a toner or astringent on a cotton wool pad, and the skin then dried with a tissue.

Peel-off masks

These are a popular form of mask and can be obtained ready prepared to suit various skin types. The manufacturer's instructions regarding use should always be followed. There are several types.

1. Gel masks

These masks may contain gelatin, gums such as tragacanth or acacia, or plastic resin, polyvinyl pyrrolidone (PVP) being particularly suitable. They may be water-based or, for quicker drying, may be alcohol-based. The preparation is applied with a brush and allowed to dry on the skin. They are easier to apply than clays, but the cleansing effect is less since gels do not absorb grease. However, they are soothing and refreshing, and make the skin feel softer since some desquamation takes place as the mask is removed. The mask shrinks during drying, tightening the skin. The film left on the skin retains body heat which increases sweating. Evaporation of the sweat is prevented, and this tends to increase the moisture content of the epidermis. The mask should be allowed to set completely, before careful removal by being peeled off in one piece.

2. Latex masks

These consist of an emulsion of rubber-based latex in water. After application to the skin, drying takes place, leaving a thin elastic film which is later removable in one piece. The film retains body heat, so promoting sweating. The skin becomes slightly filled out with moisture and slight erythema may be caused. Thus the blood supply to the skin is temporarily increased.

3. Wax masks

Wax masks consist of a mixture of beeswax, paraffin wax and petroleum jelly which is warmed to 48°C before use, preferably by using a thermostacially controlled heater. The melted wax is brushed on to the face and allowed to solidify. The warmth increases the blood supply to the skin and sweating is also increased. Skin debris sticks to the wax and is removed when the mask is peeled off the face.

Warm oil masks

A series of fine gauze masks are cut to the shape of the face, making suitable holes for the eyes, nose and mouth. These are soaked in warm olive or almond oil and applied to the face in rotation over a period of about 15 minutes, each mask being replaced by another as it cools. The eyes should be covered with dampened cotton wool pads. These masks are most useful for dry, dehydrated or crêpey skin. The oily residue is removed from the face by tissues on completion of treatment.

Questions

1. Explain how you would assess a client's skin for a suitable face pack.
2. Describe a natural face pack suitable for (a) a greasy skin and (b) a dry skin.
3. List the various types of face packs and masks, stating the beneficial effects in each case.
4. What are the contra-indications to the use of face packs and masks?
5. Describe the method of preparation, application and removal of a clay-based mask suitable for a client with sensitive skin.

Chapter 9

Eyebrow shaping

The eyebrows follow the curves of the brow bones (orbital ridges), and their function is to divert sweat from the eyes. When well-shaped, they give balance and expression to the face and will also enhance its shape. The eyebrows may often require grooming and definition, rather than an alteration to the basic natural shape.

Factors affecting eyebrow shaping

1. The shape and condition of the existing brows
The state and shape of the existing brows must be observed before commencing any treatment. If the client has been too severe in an attempt to pluck her own eyebrows and has removed too many hairs, she should be advised to let them grow in order to achieve the desired shape later. If the brows are very bushy, several sessions may be necessary before the final shape is reached. The skin around the brows is usually sensitive, and this limits the amount of plucking that can be carried out at any one time. Over-plucking may make the skin sore and inflamed. The natural line of the brows should always be followed and drastic shaping avoided, or the natural effect will be lost.

2. Fashion trends
Fashion trends often dictate changes in eyebrow shapes. These may vary from pencil slim one year to quite substantial or thick brows another year.

3. The age of the client
The client's age should always be taken into account since eyebrow shape can alter the face quite considerably. A mature client would need a flattering shape with brows which are neither too thin nor too thick. Thin brows tend to give a hard look to the face, while thick brows may make the client look older. Normal eyebrows should arch gently and should look completely natural.

4. The spacing of the eyes
Ideally, the distance between the eyes should be the width of one eye. This would, of course, be found on a perfect face. With clever eye work

the cosmetician can, however, create the illusion of perfectly spaced eyes. The effect of close-set eyes can be minimised by removing a little hair from either side of the bridge of the nose and slightly increasing the length of the brows to compensate. This creates a wider gap between the eyebrows, so giving the illusion of wider spaced eyes. Similarly, in order to make the eyes appear closer together if they are too widely spaced, the area between the eyebrows should be reduced and their length correspondingly slightly shortened.

5. *The shape of the face*

It is usual to follow the natural eyebrow shape of the client unless this is not complementary to the face shape. The eyebrows can play an extremely important part in improving the shape of a face and careful study of the client's face shape is necessary before deciding on an appropriate eyebrow shape. The client's own preferences must always be determined by consultation before carrying out a change of shape. If the shape is to be altered it should be done in such a way that it looks natural and satisfies the client's requirements.

Examples of eyebrow shapes are shown in Fig. 9.1. Almost any type of eyebrow shape is suitable for the perfect oval-shaped face.

The round face

The eyebrows are shaped in order to create an arch which will give the illusion of slimming the face.

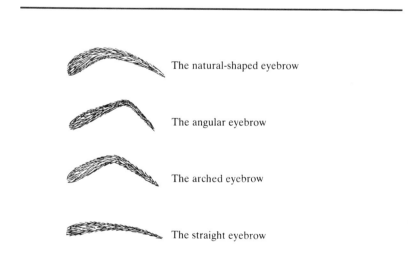

The natural-shaped eyebrow

The angular eyebrow

The arched eyebrow

The straight eyebrow

Fig. 9.1 Eyebrow shapes

The square face
The eyebrows are given an angular shape towards the outer portion of the eye which gives the illusion of rounding off the squareness of the face.

The triangular-shaped face
In order to give the appearance of a wider forehead the eyebrows should be given a well-defined arch, though this should not be too high.

The oblong face
In order to create more width and give the illusion of shortening the length of the face, the eyebrows should be kept almost straight with just the minimum of curve.

Methods of hair removal

There are several methods of hair removal but few are suitable for use around the eyes due to the sensitive nature of the skin in that area.

1. Waxing
Depilatory waxes contain a mixture of beeswax and paraffin wax and have a melting point just above normal skin temperature. The melted waxes are painted on to the skin and allowed to solidify. On stripping off the wax (in the opposite direction to the growth of the hairs), any hairs embedded in it are also removed. This method is rarely used around the eyes due to the delicacy of the tissues and the danger of warm wax entering the eye itself.

2. Razoring
This should not be used for eyebrow shaping as it results in a bristly growth of blunt cut hair, the normally tapering point having been cut away.

3. Cutting by scissors
Scissors are sometimes used to trim the bushy eyebrows of elderly men, but the method is not used for shaping.

4. Chemical depilatories
These are usually creams containing calcium thioglycollate which destroys hair by breaking down keratin. They are also capable of damaging skin keratin, and should never be used on the thin delicate skin of the eye area.

5. Electrolysis and diathermy
These methods involve the permanent removal of hair by destruction of the hair papilla. The processes are lengthy and expensive, and permanent shaping of the eyebrows is rarely thought to be advantageous.

6. Plucking

Plucking or shaping with tweezers is the most satisfactory method of shaping eyebrows. It is simple and quick and if carried out under hygienic conditions is quite safe.

To determine the correct length of the eyebrow

In order to determine the normal position of the eyebrow, an imaginary line should be drawn vertically from the edge of the nose through the inner corner of the eye to the brow (see Fig. 9.2). The eyebrow should start here. From the same point at the edge of the nose, a diagonal line is taken through the outer corner of the eye to the brow, where the eyebrow should finish. The eyebrow should follow a gentle curve with its highest point just above the outer edge of the iris. It is extremely important to follow the natural line of the eyebrow and not to attempt to alter the natural shape too drastically.

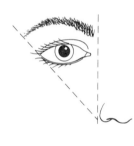

Fig. 9.2 To determine the length of the eyebrow

Equipment required for eyebrow shaping

The equipment and materials required for shaping should be prepared and placed on the trolley or left in an ultra-violet cabinet, as appropriate, before the arrival of the client.

1. Tweezers.
   There are two types of tweezers, automatic and manual (see Fig. 1.1). Automatic tweezers are spring-loaded and are ideal for removing the bulk of excess hair. Manual tweezers are used for achieving the final eyebrow shape, where a more accurate line is required. The ends of the tweezers may vary in shape from angled to square. The end shape is a matter of personal preference but, irrespective of the shape, the ends should meet perfectly without leaving any gaps. The tweezers

should be wiped with a swab of cotton wool impregnated with surgical spirit before and after shaping the eyebrows. They should always be re-sterilised after use.

2. Eyebrow brushes.
   These should be washed thoroughly after use, prior to sterilising, and kept in an ultra-violet cabinet until required.
3. Cotton wool and tissues.
4. Antiseptics (surgical spirit or cetrimide).
5. Astringent lotion or toner.

Procedure for shaping

The operator's hands must be washed before treatment is commenced. The client's requirements should be discussed and a suitable eyebrow shape chosen. The client's clothing should be protected by a towel.

Treatment

1. Cleanse the eyebrow area by wiping with a cotton wool pad dampened with astringent lotion to ensure that the area is grease-free.
2. Brush the brows first in an upward movement, and then into shape to follow the natural line.
3. Moisten two cotton wool pads with warm water and apply these to the eyebrow area. This helps to soften the tissue and will facilitate the removal of the hairs.
4. Wipe the sterilised automatic tweezers with surgical spirit and, following the prescribed guidelines, commence the shaping at the bridge of the nose.
5. Remove the warm cotton wool pads and, holding the skin firmly, pluck the hairs swiftly in the direction of their growth (see Fig. 9.3). This is the least painful method and also prevents distortion of the hair follicle which may later result in the new hair growing into the skin. Follow the natural line of the brow and work outwards, wiping the tweezers on sterile cotton wool to remove the loose hairs.
6. Work on the eyebrows alternately to ensure that they match each other both in shape and thickness. Brush them frequently in order to check the shape accurately. Only the hairs from under the brow should be plucked as otherwise the natural line will be lost.
7. If the brows become sensitive, re-apply fresh warm pads.
8. Use manual tweezers to finish the shape (see Fig. 9.4).
9. Brush the brows and at this stage consult the client on the finished result. If this is satisfactory, apply a mild astringent or an antiseptic and then rebrush the brows into their new shape.

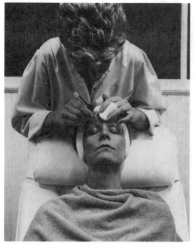

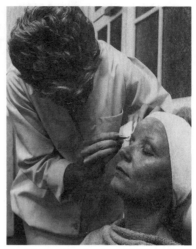

Fig. 9.3 Shaping the eyebrows with automatic tweezers

Fig. 9.4 Finishing the shape with manual tweezers

Precautions

1. The operator's hands must be clean and all equipment sterilised before commencing treatment.
2. The client must be sitting comfortably in a good light. If extra light is necessary, an angle-poise lamp may be used.
3. Razors and depilatory creams must not be used.
4. Care must be taken to avoid plucking the skin, especially when automatic tweezers are being used.
5. Hairs should not be plucked from above the brow line.
6. Contact with the eye itself must be avoided.
7. If the eyebrows have not been plucked previously, care should be taken not to be too severe at the first treatment, since the skin may be unduly sensitive. Shaping should be a gradual process carried out over a period of weeks until the final shape is achieved. Treatment should then follow every two or three weeks to maintain the shape.
8. If the client plucks her own brows, she should be advised of the correct procedure. This will avoid the disfigurement of the brows which the cosmetician may not be able to rectify until the brows have re-grown.

Contra-indications to eyebrow shaping

(a) Cuts and abrasions in the eye area.
(b) Eye disorders, e.g. conjunctivitis and styes.
(c) Inflammation or swelling of the eye area.

Questions

1. Explain the difference between automatic and manual tweezers and state the use of each.
2. Explain why razors and depilatory creams should not be used for eyebrow shaping.
3. What steps would you take if:
   (a) the brows became sensitive during plucking;
   (b) the skin were accidentally plucked when using automatic tweezers?
4. Explain why during eyebrow shaping:
   (a) hairs are plucked only from under the brow;
   (b) the brows must be brushed frequently;
   (c) cotton wool pads moistened with warm water are applied to the eyebrow area;
   (d) hairs are always plucked in the direction of growth.
5. What eyebrow shaping treatment would you advise for a client:
   (a) whose brows had not been plucked previously;
   (b) whose brows had been over-plucked;
   (c) who was elderly;
   (d) who had a very round face?

Chapter 10

Eyelash and eyebrow tinting

Tinting may be carried out on clients of any age group and is designed to give extra prominence to the brows and lashes, to blend with the client's own hair colour, and to alleviate the need for mascara, particularly for those who are allergic to it. Fair or blonde clients often require brow and lash tints to give more colour and emphasis to their usually indistinct lashes and brows.

Composition of tints

The range of colouring matter permitted in eyelash and eyebrow tints is controlled by the regulations of the EEC and the Food and Drugs Acts of this country. Certain substances such as resorcinol, pyrogallol and meta phenylenediamine, which are regarded as safe in tints for scalp hair, are not permitted in preparations intended for use in the eye area. The skin around the eye is thinner and more sensitive than that of the scalp and there is greater danger of the product entering the eye itself. For this reason, dyes formulated for use on scalp hair must never be used on the brows or lashes.

Most eyebrow and eyelash tints are mixtures of dye materials and usually include a proportion of toluenediamine. This is a permanent dye which requires oxidation before reaching its final colour. The dye base as purchased is therefore mixed with hydrogen peroxide before application to the brows or lashes. The dye molecules are small enough to enter the hair shafts, where oxidation takes place. During oxidation the dye molecules join together to form larger coloured molecules which become trapped inside the hair shafts. Since they are insoluble and too large to be washed out of the hairs, the dye is permanent.

The tints are produced in the form of liquids, creams or gels, though liquids are less popular since they are more difficult to control during application. There are several colours available including black, brown, grey, blue and auburn. Re-application of the dye is recommended at intervals of 5–7 weeks. This type of dye may produce an allergic reaction in some people, and a skin test is necessary at least 48 hours before the intended application, to ensure safe usage.

Test for allergy to the tint (predisposition or hypersensitivity test)

Cleanse an area in the fold of the elbow or behind the ear with surgical spirit using a cotton wool pad. Mix a small quantity of tint with an equal amount of 10 volumes (3 per cent) hydrogen peroxide and apply a little to the cleansed area. Allow the tint to dry, then cover with collodion and leave for 48 hours. If irritation or inflammation occurs the test will have proven positive, and under no circumstances should the treatment be carried out. The area may be treated with calamine lotion to relieve the irritation. If there is no reaction the test will have proven negative and it is safe to proceed.

Contra-indications to eyelash and eyebrow tinting

In addition to a positive reaction to the skin test, the following are also contra-indicative of tinting.
(a) Cuts and abrasions in the eye area.
(b) Eye disorders such as conjunctivitis, styes and blepharitis.
(c) Any swelling, puffiness or redness in the skin around the eye.

Preparation for tinting

1. Prepare the trolley with tint, 10 volume hydrogen peroxide, cotton wool, petroleum jelly, eye shields and previously sterilised tinting brushes or orange sticks and a spatula. An eyebath should be left in an ultra-violet cabinet in case it is required later.
2. Prior to the commencement of tinting, the client should have had a facial cleanse and tone. The eyelashes should be free from mascara and the area free from grease which may inhibit the tint.
3. The client should be gowned and seated comfortably in an almost upright position.
4. Check for any possible contra-indications.
5. Consult the client in order to choose the correct colour.
6. Wash your hands.

Tinting the eyelashes

1. Using a sterilised brush or a protected orange stick, carefully apply petroleum jelly to the skin encircling the treatment area, but avoiding contact with the lashes as this may inhibit the action of the tint.
2. Shape two damp cotton wool pads to follow the contours of the lower lid or use ready-prepared paper eye shields, and place them under the lower lashes, gently sliding them to the base of the hairs (see Fig. 10.1).

3. Mix the required amount of the chosen tint with 10 volume hydrogen peroxide, always following the manufacturer's instructions regarding correct usage. The tint should be mixed in a non-metallic dish since some metals may act as a catalyst causing immediate release of oxygen gas from hydrogen peroxide.

4. Using a clean sterilised brush or an orange stick covered with cotton wool, apply the tint to the lower lashes while the client's eyes are completely open. Work from the roots of the lashes to the tips.

5. Ask the client to close her eyes and apply the tint evenly to the upper lashes (see Fig. 10.1).

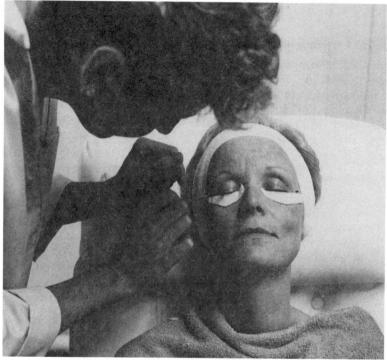

Fig. 10.1 Tinting the eyelashes

6. Apply damp cotton wool pads to the closed eyelids and allow the tint to process according to the manufacturer's instructions for 5–15 minutes.

7. Remove the pads and pad shapes in one movement and, in doing so, wipe excess tint from the lashes in an outward sweep. The client's eyes should remain closed while any remaining tint is removed with clean damp cotton wool pads.

8. When all the tint appears to have been removed, ask the client to open her eyes and check that there is none remaining at the roots. If

tint is still present, use a moistened cotton wool bud to remove it using a downwards movement while the eye is closed. Check once again with the eyes open that all excess tint has been removed.

9. Two fresh moistened cotton wool pads should be placed over the eyes and left for five minutes to help to relax them.

Tinting the eyebrows

1. Ensure that the brows are clean and grease-free and prepare them by encircling with petroleum jelly.
2. Mix a small amount of the correct colour of tint with 10 volume hydrogen peroxide according to manufacturer's instructions.
3. Using a brush or orange stick covered with cotton wool, carefully apply the tint working from the bridge of the nose to the outer edge of the brow.
4. Allow the tint to develop following the manufacturer's recommended time. The brows will usually take the colour much more rapidly than the lashes. Development time is usually between 1–2 minutes. If, after that time, the brows are not dark enough, re-apply the tint and leave for a further 1–2 minutes.
5. Remove the excess tint with damp cotton wool, working in the same direction as in the application.

Precautions in tinting

1. Always carry out a skin test 48 hours prior to the treatment, and only proceed if the test proves negative.
2. Use sterilised equipment and wash your hands before commencing application.
3. Petroleum jelly must always be used as a protection to keep the tint off the skin and avoid skin staining.
4. Tint should not be allowed to enter the client's eyes, but should it accidentally do so the tint must be removed immediately and the eye flushed out with water using a sterilised eyebath.
5. If a client is prone to blinking, apply the tint to the top lashes only. Constant blinking would make application to the lower lashes very difficult.
6. Check that all excess tint is removed, otherwise irritation may occur.
7. If the client requires an eyebrow shape in addition to an eyebrow tint, it would be wise to carry out the tint first and then the shape. Plucking may cause sensitivity which could be aggravated by the tint application. However, if there is noticeable sensitivity after the tinting of the brows, do not carry out the shape as this will cause further discomfort.
8. Avoid using too dark a tint for the eyebrows as this produces a harsh expression.

Questions

1. For what reasons do clients usually request an eyelash tint?
2. Explain the action you would take if eyelash tint accidentally entered the client's eye.
3. Explain why:
   (a) petroleum jelly is applied to encircle the treatment area before tinting the lashes or brows;
   (b) it is important to keep the petroleum jelly off the lashes and brows themselves.
4. What procedure should be adopted if a client requests an eyebrow shape and an eyebrow tint on the same occasion?
5. What precautions are necessary prior to carrying out an eyelash tint?

Chapter 11

Foundations and face shaping

In order to create a perfect make-up one would need a perfect face. This, of course, is a rarity and the cosmetician must use artistry and skill in accentuating the client's good facial features and in camouflaging any facial defects. Thus cosmetics may be used to cover skin blemishes or to change the apparent shape of the face and other facial features such as the nose and chin. The cosmetics used in face shaping are called contour cosmetics. The corrective make-up used to enhance the eyes and lips is described in Chapters 12 and 13. The success of any make-up, however, depends to a large extent on the application of the correct foundation.

Foundations

Foundations are applied to even out the natural skin tone, to form a suitable base for contour cosmetics and to provide an even surface to which powder will adhere. Modified forms of foundations may be used as blemish concealers.

Types of foundation

Foundations are available as creams, liquids, gels and cakes.

1. Creams

Originally cream foundations were untinted oil-in-water emulsions containing stearic acid (a white waxy substance) as the oil phase. On evaporation of the water from the emulsion, a fine film of tiny waxy crystals was left on the skin. These were practically invisible and the cream was known as *vanishing cream*.

Modern foundations are tinted and are usually oil-in-water emulsions containing mineral oil and ceresin wax in the oil phase. Colours vary from white to a deep mahogany to include the darker shades necessary for black skin. The creams are often coloured by use of inorganic pigments such as iron oxides which may be mined from the ground or prepared synthetically. Natural iron oxides are known by various names, e.g. ochre, sienna, burnt sienna, umber, red oxide of iron and black oxide of iron, and produce yellow, red, brown and black pigments. Titanium dioxide may be added to make a more opaque cream to increase covering power. *All-in-one bases* are mixtures of cream foundation and powder (consisting mostly of talc and kaolin), which produces a foundation with a very matt finish.

2. Liquid foundations

These may contain similar ingredients to cream foundations but have a higher proportion of water in the emulsion. Some liquid foundations are prepared without oil and are suspensions of pigments in alcohol and water, with bentonite clay added to thicken the product and hold the pigments in suspension.

Medicated foundations for acnefied skin are modified liquid foundations containing astringents and mild antiseptics such as hexachlorophene.

3. Gel foundations

Liquid foundations may also be modified by the addition of gum tragacanth or aluminium stearate to give a jelly-like consistency slightly more fluid than petroleum jelly. The gel provides a glossy film often used to produce a smooth tanned look in fashion make-up. Clear gels form suitable foundations for unblemished black skin. Gels have very little covering power.

4. Cake foundations

Emulsions containing mineral oil and carnauba wax with added pigments and powder (talc and kaolin) are dried, powdered and compressed into solid cake foundation. Cake foundations have a high covering power and are useful for covering minor blemishes.

Choice of foundation

A wide selection of foundations should be available to the cosmetician to suit varying skin types and to give a variety of colour. The foundation should ideally match the client's own skin tone although darker tones may be used on those preferring a tanned look. The correct choice of foundation as regards both texture and colour is crucial. The wrong choice could result in a shiny skin, blotchy colour or too much contrast between the natural skin tone and the foundation colour. A guide to correct foundations for different skin types is given in Table 11.1. Sug-

Table 11.1 Foundations suitable for various skin types

Skin type	Suitable foundation
Normal skin	Any type of foundation
Dry skin	Cream foundation or oil-based
Greasy skin	Liquid foundation or water-based
Combination skin	All-in-one foundation or liquid
Sensitive skin	Hypo-allergenic foundation
Blemished skin	Medicated foundation

gestions for foundation colours suitable for various skin tones are shown in Table 11.2

Table 11.2 Foundation colours for various skin tones

Skin tone	Foundation colour
Pale or fair	Light beige with warm tones of pink or peach
Medium	Warm beige or honey beige
Olive	Dark beige or bronze
Suntanned	Bronze or tan
High colour	Matt beige or foundation with a green hue
Sallow	Tan or dark beige
Light brown	Dark foundation with warm tones
Medium brown (bronzed)	Brown (all tones)
Dark brown	Golden, slightly orange gel
Black	Golden, slightly orange gel

Application of foundations

Foundations may be applied with either a damp sponge or the fingers. Cream foundations should be placed on the back of the non-working hand and liquids in the palm of the hand. The application takes place from the throat to the forehead, covering the entire face including the lips and eyelids, working methodically to achieve an even, natural finish. The hairline, creases of the nose, and the eyebrows should be checked for excess foundation causing clogging.

Translucent powder

Transluscent powder (loose powder) is used after the foundation and any cream products such as face shapers, blushers and eye shadows have been applied. If it is intended to use powdered cosmetics instead of creams, the translucent powder is applied directly on to the foundation and the powdered cosmetics used afterwards. The purpose of translucent powder is to set the make-up, to prevent shine, and to prevent the make-up from melting and moving or slipping on the skin due either to the heat of the body or the environment.

This type of powder is unpigmented or very lightly pigmented since the colour of the foundation and cream cosmetics must show through. The main ingredients are:

1. *Talc* (magnesium silicate). This forms the main bulk of the powder and consists of minute flat platelets which slide easily over each other making it very smooth.
2. *Kaolin* (aluminium silicate) which is a more absorbent substance than talc and has more covering power.
3. *Magnesium stearate* which makes the powder more adhesive and softer.
4. *Precipitated chalk* which provides bloom, giving the powder a velvety appearance on the face.

Pressed powders

These are similar to loose powders but are pressed into a cake after adding an increased amount of magnesium stearate as a binding agent. They are pigmented and usually contain titanium dioxide or zinc oxide to make them more opaque and increase their covering power. Pressed powders are designed for touching up make-up during the day, and are not suitable for 'setting' the make-up.

Application of translucent powder

Dip a clean ball of cotton wool into the powder once and then apply it to the face from a clean tissue placed in the palm of the non-working hand. Press the cotton wool gently but firmly over the entire foundation. Using a sterilised powder brush, remove excess powder by brushing first upwards against the facial hair and then downwards following the natural lie of the hair. The client's eyes should remain closed throughout the powder application. Should more powder be required from the container, always use a clean ball of cotton wool.

If the matt effect created by the powder is not required, press a slightly dampened piece of cotton wool lightly over the face to produce a translucent effect.

Precautions in use

1. Work quickly and methodically.
2. Do not allow powder to enter the client's eyes or mouth.
3. Rebrush the eyebrows after the application to remove any excess powder.
4. Check the whole application for excess loose powder.

Contra-indications to use

1. Excessively dry skin.
2. Excessive facial hair.

Contour cosmetics

These are cosmetics which are used either to shade or to highlight particular features of the face. They can emphasise or subdue a feature depending on where they are used and also on the colour chosen. The cosmetician must be skilful in the use of contour cosmetics in order to achieve good balance, shape and design when carrying out a make-up. When correctly used, contour cosmetics can help to create the illusion of the perfect oval face.

Contour cosmetics include *highlighters*, *shaders* and *blushers* (rouge) and all are available as both creams or powders. They differ basically in colour and use. Highlighters are light coloured (white, cream or beige) and are used to emphasise good facial features. Shaders are dark toned (usually shades of brown) and are used to subdue facial defects by creating shadows or hollows. Blushers are designed to add colour (pink, peach and various shades of red) usually to accentuate the cheek bones and give warmth to the skin.

Types of contour cosmetics

1. Cream products

Cream highlighters, shaders and blushers may be oil-in-water emulsions but are more usually non-aqueous mixtures of mineral oils, petroleum jelly, and waxes such as beeswax or carnauba wax. In less greasy products, isopropyl myristate and ozokerite may replace some of the mineral oil. Powder (kaolin and talc) may also be added. They are coloured by use of inorganic pigments, usually some form of iron oxide to give brown shades, or by insoluble lakes which produce a range of brighter colours. Lakes are formed when soluble coal tar dyes are treated with metallic hydroxides such as aluminium hydroxide.

2. Powder products

These contain the same ingredients as translucent powder though they are more highly tinted and have an increased amount of magnesium stearate, which acts as a binder so that the powder can be successfully pressed into a cake. They are coloured by inorganic pigments or lakes. Titanium dioxide, an intensely white substance, may be added to make the powder more opaque.

Use of foundations as contour cosmetics

If contour cosmetics are not available, foundations may be adapted for use as highlighters and shaders. A foundation selected for highlighting must be two shades lighter than the shade of the base foundation which is used over the entire face. For use as a shader, a foundation must be two shades darker than the base shade.

Application of contour cosmetics

1. Contour cosmetic creams are applied by dotting the cream where required on the face or eyelids, and blending it in with the finger tips. Powder products are applied with a sterilised brush. To avoid spoiling the make-up already applied, a tissue may be used to ensure that the hands do not come into contact with the face.
2. Whenever contour cosmetics are used, it is essential that they blend into the foundation in order to prevent harsh lines of demarcation between one cosmetic and another.

3. The over-emphasis of facial hair should be avoided when using shaders.
4. Blushers should be kept away from the eyes and nose, and should always be blended in with an upwards movement.
5. Subtle use of contour cosmetics is necessary to keep the make-up looking as natural as possible.
6. The application should be checked on completion to ensure that it is symmetrical.

The shape of the face

Before contour cosmetics are used it is important that the cosmetician examines the client's face both from the front and in profile, to determine the shape of the face, nose and chin, and to note the length and width of the neck. Face shape largely depends on the formation of the bones of the face, and on the amount of muscle and subcutaneous fat in the cheeks and on the chin. The presence of well-formed cheek muscles tends to produce a rounder face, but in older people the sagging of these muscles may change the contours to give a squarer jaw line (hence the need for face lifting which involves the raising of the cheek muscles).

For Europeans there are seven basic face shapes (oval, round, heart-shaped, square, oblong, diamond and triangular) though some faces are a mixture of these. The bone structure corresponding to the seven shapes is shown in Fig. 11.1.

The facial features of some African and Asian clients may not be compatible with the division into seven basic face shapes, since the whole bone structure and depth of the face may be different. The black African may have high cheekbones which lend themselves to highlighting and blusher. The jaw is usually prominent and emphasises the larger mouth shape and full lips, while the nasal bones tend to be flatter. Highlighting is often more effective than shading on black skin since the darker colours required for shading do not show up well.

Asian faces vary considerably but are usually flatter and may be oval or round. Greater emphasis is usually paid to eye make-up including the striking use of kohl eyeliner. Chinese faces are often round with broad flat noses, small almond-shaped eyes and full lips.

Ideas of beauty also vary and, when dealing with African and Asian clients, the cosmetician must discuss the requirements carefully. The basic principles of highlighting and shading still apply, though differently coloured products may be required. Each face must be treated individually.

Corrective face shaping

The aim of face shaping is to carry out corrective work to improve the overall shape of the face by creating the illusion of an oval shape using highlighting and shading techniques.

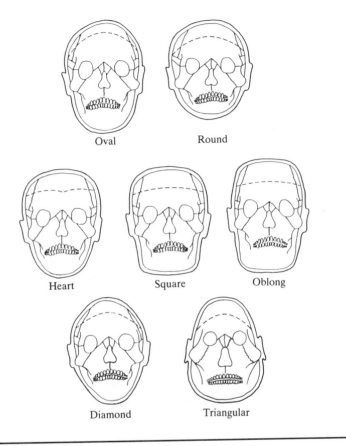

Fig. 11.1 Face shapes (bone structure)

The oval face
This is recognised as the ideal face shape and all styles of make-up look good on this type (see Fig. 11.2).

The round face
This face is short and broad with full rounded cheeks. Shading the side of the cheeks gives the appearance of a more slender face (see Fig. 11.3).

The heart-shaped face
A heart-shaped face has a characteristically wide forehead with the face narrowing to the jawline. Highlighting the jawline creates the appearance of width while the breadth of the forehead is reduced by shading (see Fig. 11.4).

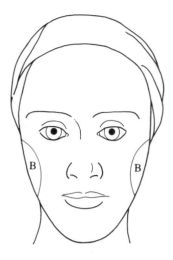

Fig. 11.2 The oval face

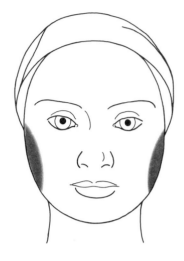

Fig. 11.3 Corrective make-up for the round face

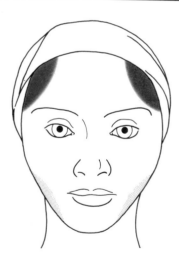

Fig. 11.4 Corrective work for the heart-shaped face

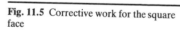

Fig. 11.5 Corrective work for the square face

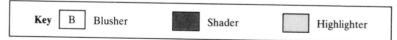

| Key | B | Blusher | | Shader | | Highlighter |

The square face
This face has an angular jawline and a correspondingly wide forehead, with full cheeks. The corners of the face are shaded to reduce the width and round off the angular lines (see Fig. 11.5).

The oblong face
The oblong face is long and narrow. The forehead and chin are shaded to reduce the length, and the sides of the face highlighted to create width (see Fig. 11.6).

The diamond-shaped face
This face is characterised by its wide cheek bones and tapering forehead and jawline. The sides of the forehead and jawline are highlighted to reduce the apparent width of the face and the chin is shaded to shorten the appearance of the face (see Fig. 11.7).

The triangular face (pear-shaped)
The triangular face has a characteristically wide jawline which tapers up to a narrow forehead. The corners of the jawline are shaded to reduce the width, and the forehead highlighted to give it a wider appearance (see Fig. 11.8).

Corrective work for nose shapes

Large prominent nose
This can be made to look smaller by applying dark foundation or shader to the nose and highlighting the surrounding area with a lighter foundation (see Fig. 11.9). The foundations must be blended evenly to avoid a demarcation line between the two. Blusher should be kept well away from the nose.

Broad nose
To give the nose a narrower appearance, the sides of the nostrils are shaded without blending the shader on to the face itself (see Fig. 11.10).

Short or flat nose (snub nose)
This nose may be given a more prominent appearance by the application of a thin strip of highlighter down its length (see Fig. 11.11).

Thin short nose
To give this nose apparent length and breadth, highlighter is applied down its length, carefully blending it on to the sides and merging it with a darker foundation on the cheeks (see Fig. 11.12).

Long nose
To give a wider effect, highlighter is applied down the centre of the nose to just above the tip which is then shaded (see Fig. 11.13).

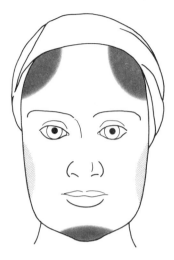

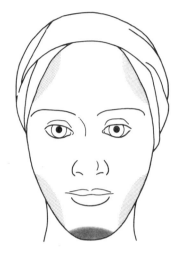

Fig. 11.6 Corrective work for the oblong face

Fig. 11.7 Corrective work for the diamond-shaped face

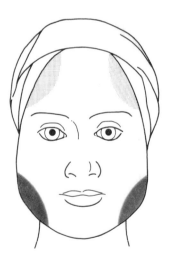

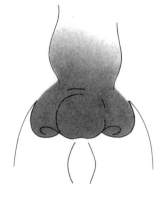

Fig. 11.8 Corrective work for the triangular face

Fig. 11.9 Corrective work for a prominent nose

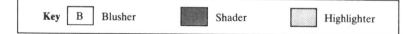

| Key | B | Blusher | | Shader | | Highlighter |

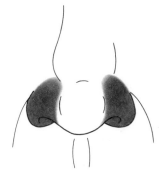

Fig. 11.10 Corrective work for a broad nose

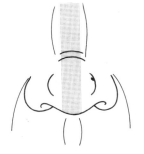

Fig. 11.11 Corrective work for a snub nose

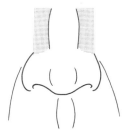

Fig. 11.12 Corrective work for a thin, short nose

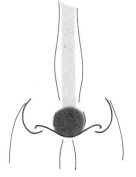

Fig. 11.13 Corrective work for a long nose

Key | B | Blusher   Shader   Highlighter

Corrective work for chins

The double chin
A double chin is characterised by folds of skin under the chin. The effect may be minimised by shading into the folds and highlighting above the jaw bone.

The protruding chin and receding chin
To lessen the prominence of the chin, a dark foundation or shader should be applied. Highlighters or lighter foundations will give the opposite effect and should therefore be applied to a receding chin.

Corrective work for the neck and jawline

It is essential when carrying out a make-up to ensure an even coverage and careful blend of foundations over the length of the face and into the neckline. This will avoid any stark contrast between the natural skin tone and the foundation.

If the neck is thick it should be shaded to slim its appearance; a thin neck should be highlighted to give a fuller appearance. The jawline may be treated in the same way. A dark foundation or shader applied to the jawline and blended up to the temples will give balance to a broad jaw, whereas a narrow jaw should be highlighted to give width.

The concealment of blemishes

Highlighters, foundations, concealer cream, blemish sticks and green corrective cream may be used in the concealment of blemishes. Concealer products are always used before the foundation is applied. They should be used sparingly and should be easily covered by the foundation itself.

Concealer cream is a coloured foundation cream containing powder (talc and kaolin), and varies in consistency according to the amount of cover required. It may be quite dense and putty-like. Thick concealer creams should be used sparingly, and are not suitable for covering large areas. The creams are usually available in various shades of beige.

Concealer sticks contain similar ingredients to concealer creams but include a higher proportion of waxes. A typical concealer stick may contain 55 per cent powder (talc and kaolin) and pigments (iron oxides and titanium dioxide), with 44 per cent of mineral oils and waxes, together with 1 per cent of water. They are usually available in white and various shades of beige. Cover sticks are sometimes required to even out the colour of black skin before make-up.

Green corrective creams are coloured foundation creams containing a green pigment such as chromium oxide, or a green lake. They are designed to disguise any unwanted redness of the face, as the green pigment will absorb any red light and prevent its reflection from blemishes on the surface of the skin.

Concealment of age lines
It is usual for most faces to develop age lines or facial expression lines. Laughter lines (crow's feet) around the eyes may be masked by applying a highlighter sparingly in the lined area: this helps to fill out the crevices. The naso-labial folds, extending from the nostrils to the corners of the mouth, may be treated in the same way by applying highlighter along the crease line before the foundation.

Concealment of dark circles under the eyes
Dark circles may be caused by lack of sleep, the ageing process or kidney malfunction. They may be concealed by applying a lighter foundation than that intended as the base shade. Concealer creams may also be used, but should be applied sparingly and confined to the hollow under the eyes.

Concealment of minor blemishes
Small scars, moles and freckles are often adequately camouflaged by foundation cream. Alternatively, a blemish stick toning with the foundation may be used. The concealer must be taken from the stick using a sterilised spatula before application to the skin. It must not be applied too thickly or it may show through the foundation.

Concealment of high colouring and broken capillaries
High colouring of the cheeks or nose, due to constant exposure to the elements or to broken capillaries, may be reduced by the use of green corrective cream. This should be dotted on to the skin using the finger tips, before applying the foundation.

Questions

1. Explain the meaning of 'contour cosmetics' and describe their uses.
2. Describe the condition known as 'crow's feet'. Explain how this condition arises and how it should be treated during make-up.
3. What is the purpose of using a foundation? What procedure should be adopted in selecting the correct foundation?
4. When and for what reason would the following be used during make-up?
   (a) a green corrective cream;
   (b) a medicated foundation;
   (c) translucent powder.
5. Why should translucent powder be avoided on clients with excessive facial hair?

Chapter 12

Eye make-up

Eye make-up may be used to accentuate the eyes, correct faults and generally to add colour to the face. The colours selected should ideally blend with those of the client's clothes and enhance the appearance of the rest of the make-up. A good eyebrow shape is essential as straggly eyebrows spoil the effect of eye make-up. Cosmetic preparations for the eyes include eye shadow, eyeliner, mascara and eyebrow pencil. Since the skin around the eyes is very thin, the eye area is particularly sensitive and all substances used in eye make-up must be of a high degree of purity.

Eye shadow

Eye shadow is used to add colour and give dimension to the eyes. Numerous colours are available, the most popular for mature clients being shades of blue, green and brown. Younger clients tend to follow fashion trends and the colours used can vary from violet through to yellow and orange. The colouring matter must be non-toxic and non-irritant, so that only certain substances are permissible by the regulations of the EEC and the Food and Drugs acts of this country. These include inorganic pigments such as those listed in Table 12.1, and some lakes made by treating soluble coal tar dyes with metallic hydroxides to render the dyes insoluble.

Lighter shades or pastel shades are obtained by adding white titanium dioxide to the pigments. For evening wear, glitter in the form of finely divided metals such as gold leaf, aluminium and bronze is sometimes

Table 12.1 Inorganic pigments used in eye make-up

Colour of make-up	Pigment used
Black	Carbon black or black iron oxide with ultramarine to give a blue-black
Grey	Lamp black, ultramarine and titanium dioxide
Brown	Mixture of iron oxides (sienna and ochre)
Red	Red iron oxide
Yellow	Yellow ochre
Green	Chromium oxide
Blue	Ultramarine
Violet	Ultramarine and carmine lake

added to eye shadow. They may also be pearlised or frosted by the addition of bismuth oxychloride (either synthetically produced or obtained from fish scales), or by the addition of mica (found as small glittering scales in granite rocks). The cosmetician should use frosted shadows with caution since they tend to accentuate the crêpeyness in the skin of a mature client, while looking vibrant and attractive on youthful skin.

Eye shadows are available in the form of powders, creams and gels.

1. Powder eye shadows

Powder eye shadows are the type most commonly used today. They contain a high proportion of talc with finely powdered pigments and a little mineral oil, pressed into a cake using magnesium stearate to bind the ingredients together.

2. Cream eye shadows

These are prepared by blending the desired pigments either in an emulsion or, more commonly, in a non-aqueous mixture of oils and waxes. The latter include mineral oil, lanolin, petroleum jelly, and microcrystalline waxes such as ozokerite and ceresin which make the cream solid in the container but liquid on contact with the skin. Replacing some of the mineral oil by isopropyl myristate makes a less greasy product.

3. Gel eye shadows

Gel eye shadows are usually suspensions of pigments in water, thickened by methyl cellulose to a jelly-like consistency. They tend to give gloss rather than depth of colour and several coats may be required to produce satisfactory cover.

Application of eye shadows

Eye shadows may be used on the entire upper lid and extended up to the brow line, and also below the lower lashes and around the eye. The cosmetician will experiment a good deal in order to develop designs or patterns for the eyelids. Strips of colour may be used in horizontal, diagonal or vertical lines depending on the effect desired. When using more than one colour on the eyelid, subtle blending is necessary to avoid the appearance of hard blocks of colour across the lid. Extreme care should always be taken when working around the eye to avoid damage to the delicate and sensitive skin of that area. The client's eyes should be closed throughout the application.

The cosmetician should always prepare a palette with a selection of the colours to be used. This avoids the unhygienic practice of dipping fingers, brushes or sponge type applicators in and out of containers, and prevents cross-infection. A sterilised palette is used and the shadows are removed from their containers on to the palette by means of a sterilised spatula.

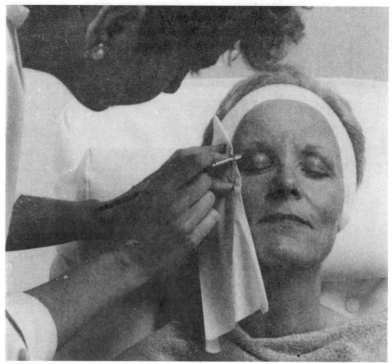

Fig. 12.1 Application of eye shadow

They are applied to the face by means of a sterilised eye make-up brush or a sponge type applicator. A tissue should be held under or near to the eyes to prevent accidental spillage from spoiling the make-up already applied (see Fig. 12.1).

Eyeliner

Eyeliner may be used to give extra prominence to the eyes. When used skilfully, the apparent size or shape of the eye can be altered.

Eyeliner is obtainable in pencil, liquid and cake form. Pencils tend to be most popular because their effect is more subtle, while liquid and cake eyeliners often give a hard look. The available colours include black and various shades of brown, blue, green, pink and violet. The pigments used to create these are the same as for eye shadows.

1. Eyeline pencils

These contain a suitable blend of oils and waxes to give a soft waxy pencil. The ingredients include mineral oil, lanolin, cetyl alcohol, petroleum jelly, beeswax, carnauba wax and ozokerite.

2. Liquid eyeliner

Liquid eyeliner consists of pigments suspended in water and thickened by gums, resins such as polyvinyl pyrrolidone, or methyl cellulose. It should be applied with a sterilised brush.

3. Cake eyeliner

This is similar to cake shadow and contains mixtures of talc, mineral oils and pigment with magnesium stearate used to bind the ingredients when pressed into a cake.

Application of eyeliner

Eyeliner is applied from the inner to the outer corner of the closed upper lid close to the roots of the eyelashes, and similarly to the under side of the lower lashes. It may also be applied to the rim of the lower lid near to the roots, in which case extreme care must be taken to avoid contact with the eyeball. Application to the lower lid can be carried out more easily if the client is asked to look upwards. Cake liner is applied from a palette using a damp brush. Pencils should be sharpened to create a clean surface before use and kept in an ultra-violet cabinet until required.

Kohl pencil

Kohl pencils are used to define the shape of the eyes and are used on the inner rim of the lids to accentuate the whites. A steady hand is required to avoid touching the eyeball itself. Kohl application is popular with young people and many eastern clients. It is usually used with a lot of eye shadow as the rim around the eyelids tends to make the eyes appear smaller. Kohl consists of black antimony sulphide and is made into pencil form by the addition of various waxes.

Mascara

Traditionally, mascara was used only to darken the eyelashes and colours were limited to black and brown, but it is now also available in shades of blue, green and pink. Fashion will dictate which colours are most popular at any given time. Mature clients tend to be conservative with regard to colour choice and invariably choose black, brown or blue. The pigments used are the same as those for eye shadows.

Mascara is available in cake, cream or liquid form.

1. Cake mascara

This consists of a mixture of mineral oil, lanolin, and waxes such as beeswax and carnauba wax, along with triethanolamine stearate (a soap). These are melted together and pressed into a cake. Silicone oils are sometimes added to improve the spread of the product. Carnauba wax acts as a water repellant. This type of mascara is applied using a moist sterilised brush. The moisture causes an emulsion to be formed at the point of contact with the cake, the triethanolamine soap acting as an emulsifying agent so that the mascara is applied as an emulsion. Cake mascara is the most suitable type for salon use, since the brush used for application is easily washed and sterilised.

2. Cream mascara

This is formulated as a pigmented oil-in-water emulsion, the oil phase containing mineral oil, lanolin, and waxes such as beeswax or carnauba wax. Triethanolamine stearate is used as the emulsifying agent since it is less alkaline than other soaps and therefore less irritant. Cream mascara is greasier than the cake type and is not as frequently used.

3. Liquid mascara

Liquid mascara usually consists of a suspension of pigments in water or in alcohol and water, thickened with methyl cellulose or with a synthetic resin such as polyvinyl acetate. A little castor oil may be added to soften the film left on the lashes after the evaporation of the water and alcohol. The use of resins produces a more waterproof product which is very popular. Short filaments of rayon or nylon may also be added to liquid mascara, these adhere to the lashes, making them appear longer and thicker. Lash extenders should not be used by contact lens wearers since the fine fibres may produce irritation if any become trapped behind the lenses. Liquid mascara is often packaged in a container equipped with its own spiral brush applicator. This type of applicator is unsuitable for salon use since it is constantly re-inserted into the container during the application and may result in cross-infection.

Application of mascara

Cake mascara is applied to the eyelashes using a moistened sterilised brush, after first transferring a little mascara from the cake on to a palette. The application involves a downward sweep over the top lashes and then an upward sweep under the same lashes, to encourage them to curve upwards. After protecting the skin by placing a tissue under the lower lashes, the mascara is applied to them with a downwards stroke. This is made easier if the client is asked to look upwards. If more than one coat of mascara is to be applied to give extra emphasis, it is important that each application is allowed to dry before proceeding with the next. This avoids clogging of the lashes or an unduly thick-looking application. Over-use of mascara should be avoided otherwise the lashes will appear too heavy. The lashes must remain separate after the application and should not adhere to each other.

Eyebrow pencils

Eyebrow pencils are used to give extra definition and colour to the eyebrows. The colours are limited to black, brown and grey. Pigments similar to those used in eye shadows are dispersed in a wax and oil base to give a firm but non-brittle wax crayon or pencil. Suitable ingredients include mineral oils, lanolin, cetyl alcohol, beeswax, ozokerite and petroleum jelly.

Application of eyebrow pencil

The eyebrows should first be brushed into shape. The eyebrow pencil should be applied using fine feathery strokes, as opposed to hard strong lines, in order to give a more natural appearance to the brow. Pencils and crayons should be sharpened before use and kept in an ultra-violet cabinet until required.

Corrective eye make-up

Eye make-up can be used to draw attention to good eye features or subdue undesirable features, and also to improve the apparent shape of the eyes. The use of dark-coloured eye shadow tends to make the eyes appear smaller while the bright colours give prominence.

Small eyes

The eyes may be made to look larger by the use of a light-coloured eye shadow on the brow bone. The centre lid may be accentuated with a softly contrasting shade extending beyond the corner of the eyes to reach the brow bone (see Fig. 12.2). A good eyebrow shape will give more space and help to enlarge the appearance of the eyes. A liberal application of mascara may be used to advantage.

Round eyes

The appearance of length can be given by extending the shadow beyond the corner of the eye. The socket line can be emphasised with a deeper shade and the brow bone highlighted (see Fig. 12.3). Mascara is best applied from the centre of the lashes outwards.

Close-set eyes

These may be improved by keeping lighter-coloured shadows near the bridge of the nose, and using a strong colour winging upwards and outwards towards the brow bone which may itself be highlighted (see Fig. 12.4). Mascara may be applied from the centre lashes and outwards.

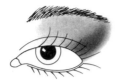

Fig. 12.2 Corrective work for small eyes

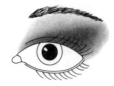

Fig. 12.3 Corrective work for round eyes

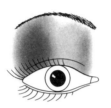

Fig. 12.4 Corrective work for close-set eyes

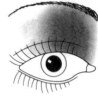

Fig. 12.5 Corrective work for wide-set eyes

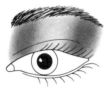

Fig. 12.6 Corrective work for narrow eyes

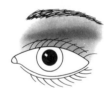

Fig. 12.7 Corrective work for deep-set eyes

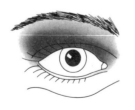

Fig. 12.8 Corrective work for protruding eyes

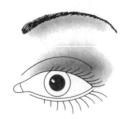

Fig. 12.9 Corrective work for hanging lids

Wide-set eyes

The use of deeper, stronger colours near the bridge of the nose blending out softly to the outer corners will give the illusion of bringing the eyes closer together (see Fig. 12.5).

Narrow eyes

Applying a light colour right down the centre of the lid from the brow to the lashes and blending a darker colour to the inner and outer corners will make the eyes appear more open and give the illusion of largeness (see Fig. 12.6).

Deep-set eyes

The use of a soft pale colour on the lid will appear to bring the eyes forwards. A deeper shade should be used to create an artificial socket line slightly above the natural line. The brow bone should be highlighted to give it prominence (see Fig. 12.7).

Protruding eyes

To minimise the protrusion, a deep shade is applied to the upper lid taking this upwards and outwards to the brow bone which is itself then highlighted to draw attention from the protrusion (see Fig. 12.8).

Hanging lids

Highlights are used from the inner corner of the eye following the socket line, with a deep matt shadow on the lid to mask its prominence (see Fig. 12.9). If a more definite appearance is required, stronger shades along the lash line must be applied.

Eye make-up for users of contact lenses

It is essential to avoid greasy preparations around the eyes if contact lenses are worn, since oil getting between the eye and the lens would blur the vision. It is usual to ask the client to remove the lenses before carrying out a make-up. If they have not been removed, the eyes should be closed when using face powder or powdered eye shadows to avoid particles adhering to them. Only waterproof mascara should be used because of the possibility of the eyes watering and causing the mascara to run. Eyelash tinting would reduce the necessity for mascara.

Eye make-up for wearers of glasses

Before make-up is attempted, note the colour of the frames, the area covered by the lenses and whether or not they are tinted. It is usual to use more colour and mascara on clients who wear glasses. Eye shadow should be chosen to complement the colour of the frames. If tinted glasses are worn, the colour of the make-up applied to the eye area would appear more subdued. It may thus be necessary to use stronger colours, e.g. deeper blue or green colours. Black mascara should also be used. False eyelashes may be used but should be short to avoid touching the lenses.

Contra-indications to the use of eye make-up

(a) Allergy to eye cosmetics.
(b) Cuts and abrasions in the eye area.
(c) Inflammation of the skin around the eye.
(d) Eye disorders, e.g. conjunctivitis and styes.

Questions

1. Describe three different cosmetics which may be used around the eyes and state the use of each.
2. What precautions are necessary when carrying out an eye make-up on a client who wears contact lenses?
3. Which eye make-up products are best suited to an elderly client? Give reasons for your answer.
4. How should eyeliner be applied to the upper lid? What effect would this have on the appearance of the eyes?
5. Discuss the precautions which must be taken to prevent cross-infection when using different types of eye make-up.

Chapter 13

Lip make-up

Lip cosmetics include lipsticks, lip pencils and lip gloss. Lipstick has always been one of the most popular cosmetics and many people who are normally averse to make-up will still use lipstick. The main purpose of lipstick is of course to impart colour to the lips, but it is also used to accentuate a good lip shape or to disguise defects and to prevent cracking and dryness.

Lipstick

Lipstick may be formulated in stick form or as a cream or liquid. The stick type consists of suitable colouring matter dispersed in a lipstick base of blended oils and waxes, which are designed to soften on contact with the lips. Lipsticks are often highly perfumed to mask the fatty odour of the base, and may also be flavoured since taste as well as smell is important in the mouth area. The traditional base contained castor oil and beeswax, but castor oil is now rarely used since it is subject to rancidity and has an unpleasant taste and odour. Modern lipsticks contain a mixture of waxes such as carnauba wax, candelilla wax, ceresin and ozokerite which gives hardness to the product, together with softer substances such as lanolin, petroleum jelly, mineral oils and isopropyl myristate. Silicone waxes may be added to improve the spreading properties of the lipstick. The proportion of waxes and the softer substances is varied according to the product required, either a firm stick containing more waxes or a soft cream containing more oils. The ingredients may also be varied to give a glossy appearance to the lips or a matt effect. Pearlised lipstick gives a softer look and contains either mica or bismuth oxychloride which increase the reflection of light from the surface of the lips.

Stick products should have a smooth surface of uniform colour, and should maintain the same consistency throughout their usable life without becoming hard and brittle or soft and flaky. On the lips the film should adhere well and not rub off during eating and drinking. It should be harmless both on the skin and if ingested with food.

Liquid lipstick may be water-based or water/alcohol-based with appropriate colouring matter and thickened with gums or methyl cellulose.

Lipstick colourings

The colour range of lipstick is extremely varied, from the palest pink through deep red to coffee and chocolate. Two types of colouring matter are used together in lipstick:

1. *Staining colours* which slightly penetrate the outer surface of the lip giving a semi-permanent colour, contain bromo-acid dyes including eosin which is most frequently used to give a bright red colour. Some clients may develop a sensitivity to this dye resulting in inflammation, cracking or peeling of the lips, and sometimes swelling and blistering of the lip tissue. Photo-sensitivity, that is allergy arising from the action of ultra-violet rays in sunlight on the dye, is also possible.
2. *Inorganic pigments* such as iron oxides, and metallic lakes are used as non-staining colours in lipsticks. The lakes, which are soluble coal tar dyes rendered insoluble by treatment with aluminium or calcium compounds, are most often used since they produce brighter colours than the pigments. For pastel shades, white titanium dioxide is added.

Hypo-allergenic lipstick

Known sensitisers such as eosin dye and lanolin are omitted from hypo-allergenic lipstick. No perfume is included and other ingredients are highly purified, e.g. beeswax may be de-pollinated.

Application of lipstick

Lipstick is applied using a sterilised lip brush (see Fig. 13.1) by first outlining the lips and then in-filling. The application should be blotted with a tissue to remove excess and then a second coat applied. The use of a brush ensures a better outline shape and a more even application of colour. In order to prevent cross-infection, a sterilised spatula is drawn across the lipstick to remove the required amount. This is then applied directly to the lips using the brush. Liquid lipstick is applied from a sterilised palette, again using a brush. During application, the skin should be protected by a tissue to avoid smudging the foundation.

The colour of the lipstick should be chosen to tone with the rest of the colours on the face and with the clothing, to give a balanced and complementary effect. Blue-toned lipstick should be avoided for clients with a florid complexion or broken capillaries; yellow and orange shades are unsuitable for sallow skins. Black clients suit dark red, brick red and purple lipsticks.

Lip pencils

These are prepared from similar ingredients to lipstick but with a higher proportion of hard waxes such as carnauba wax to make a wax crayon.

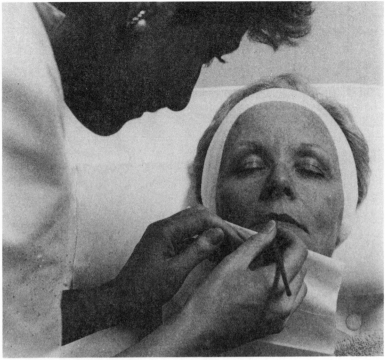

Fig. 13.1 Application of lipstick

Lip pencils are often used to line the outer edge of the lips before the application of lipstick of a complementary colour. To ensure the hygienic use of lip pencils and avoid cross-infection, they should be sharpened to create a clean surface and then sterilised before re-use.

Lip gloss or gel

Lip gloss, as its name implies, is used to give a lustrous and glossy appearance to lips. It may be colourless or tinted and contains mineral oils made to a gel consistency by the addition of bentonite clay which also suspends any pigments used. The gel is applied over the lipstick using a sterilised brush. This type of product has a tendency to wear off quickly and, if tinted, gives only a minimum of colour.

Corrective lip shaping

Well made-up, clearly defined lips will complement the whole make-up and give added interest to the face. Any slight defect in the shape of the lips can be corrected by the skilful use of lipstick and lip pencil. Dark colours tend to make the lips look smaller, and light colours to make them appear larger.

Thin lips

These can be made to appear fuller by pencilling just outside the natural line though still following the original curves, before filling in with lipstick (see Fig. 13.2).

Full lips

The appearance of full lips may be slimmed by carefully pencilling in a new line slightly inside the natural one but following the original curve, before filling in with lipstick (see Fig. 13.3).

Unbalanced lips

If the top lip is thinner than the lower lip, extra fullness can be added to the upper lip by pencilling in a new bow slightly above the existing one and then filling in the new shape. If the lower lip is the thinner of the two, the shape should be extended slightly below the existing line. In each case the new line should be kept within the outer borders of the mouth, as otherwise an unnatural hard look will result (see Fig. 13.4).

Asymmetrical mouth

In this case one side of the top lip is narrower than the other. This may be corrected by carefully pencilling slightly above the narrow side to give balance (see Fig. 13.5).

Drooping mouth

This type of mouth gives an impression of sadness which may be counteracted by building up the corners of the lower lip line to meet the upper lip line (see Fig. 13.6).

The ageing mouth

Vertical lines appear around the mouth with age, particularly if the teeth have been removed, and the lips lose their clearly defined outline. Smokers tend to develop a prematurely lined mouth. The use of greasy lipsticks or pencils should be avoided as 'bleeding' may occur into the fine lines. This results in loss of the original shape which will in turn spoil the whole make-up. The lips should be outlined with a dry lip pencil and lip gloss kept to a minimum.

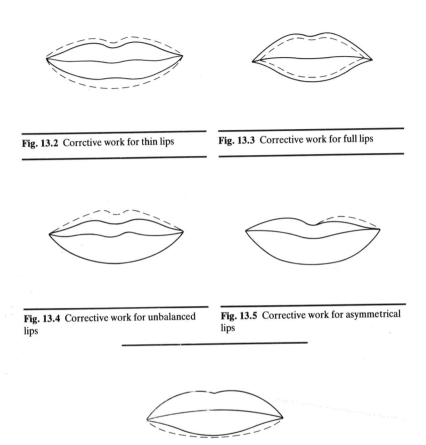

Fig. 13.2 Corrective work for thin lips

Fig. 13.3 Corrective work for full lips

Fig. 13.4 Corrective work for unbalanced lips

Fig. 13.5 Corrective work for asymmetrical lips

Fig. 13.6 Corrective work for a drooping mouth

Contra-indications to lip cosmetics

(a) Allergy to lip cosmetics.
(b) Infections in the area of the mouth, e.g. cold sores or impetigo.

Questions

1. Explain why lipstick is best applied with a lip brush.

2. How may cross-infection be avoided when using (a) a lipstick and (b) a lip pencil?
3. Why should greasy lipstick be avoided for elderly clients?
4. State three qualities which are required in a good lipstick.
5. State the possible reasons for using (a) a dark lipstick and (b) a light-coloured lipstick.

Chapter 14

Day and evening make-up

Make-up can make or mar a face. The skill and artistic ability of the cosmetician in the use of cosmetics should result in the creation of an attractive face, but it is important also that the client herself is comfortable and confident with the finished result. The salon environment in which the make-up is carried out should be serene and completely hygienic.

Before carrying out any work it is essential that the cosmetician observes the shape of the client's face and facial features, the skin tone, hair colour and any blemishes and facial hair which may be present. The client's age and personality will also affect the type of make-up worn. The client should always be consulted with regard to her personal preferences and the occasion for which the make-up is required.

Day make-up

Day make-ups are the most difficult to perfect since the final effect should be subtle and completely natural looking. Make-up should therefore be light and under- rather than over-used.

Evening make-up

Evening make-up is by convention more adventurous than day make-up mainly because certain colours, especially shades of grey and brown, are not clearly seen in subdued artificial light and so much brighter colours are often required. Cosmetics specifically used for evening wear include glitter, gold and silver eye make-up, lip gloss and false eyelashes. If more prominence is required for the eyes, the client should be advised to have her lashes tinted beforehand. The make-up must be adapted according to the occasion or function for which it is intended, and also to the clothing to be worn. The application must be skilfully carried out so that the client does not feel too conspicuous, especially if she is not used to wearing a lot of make-up. It should be explained to the client that the evening make-up may appear much brighter in natural daylight but will be more subdued under artificial light.

Fantasy make-up

Fantasy make-up can be used for evening wear but is usually worn only by the younger client. This type of make-up is often used competitively when a 'total look' is required. (A 'total look' means the entire make-up and costume or dress, and usually depicts a particular theme.) Stencils may be used but extreme care should be taken to ensure that the design on the face is compatible with the costume or the image the client wishes to create, otherwise the effect will be lost and may look decidedly odd. It may help to work out the design and colour scheme on paper before attempting it on the face.

Lighting

During make-up the client should be well illuminated with the light falling directly on to her face, so that no shadows are cast on the face itself. The source of light is also important since the colour of cosmetics is affected by the colour of the light falling on them. When we talk about the colour of an object we normally mean its colour in 'white' light (that is, in daylight or sunlight). If sunlight passes through a glass prism (see Fig. 14.1) it may be split up into a band of colour known as a spectrum which consists of the seven colours red, orange, yellow, green, blue, indigo and violet. Thus white light consists of light of these seven colours in the proportion produced in the spectrum.

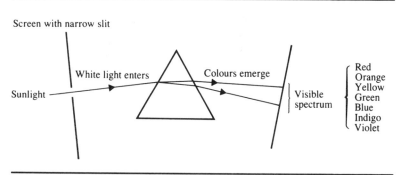

Fig. 14.1 The spectrum

The molecules of pigment or dye in an object will absorb certain colours of light and reflect others. The colours which are reflected to our eyes determine the colour we 'see'. If white light falls on a red lipstick, the pigment in the lipstick reflects the red light to our eyes and absorbs the other six colours; the lipstick therefore appears red. However, if pure blue light falls on the lipstick it will be absorbed and since there is no red light for it to reflect the lipstick will appear black. Similarly, clothes and the skin appear to change colour when viewed under yellow 'sodium' street lamps or under the constantly changing coloured lights at a disco.

The colour of light produced artificially by electric filament lamps or by fluorescent tubes is different from that of daylight and so changes the apparent colour of objects. Thus make-up to be worn in daylight is best applied in daylight or, if this is impossible, a 'daylight' type fluorescent lamp would give a similar effect. Filament lamps produce light containing more red and yellow light and less blue and green than is found in daylight. Thus they tend to make red colours appear deeper and blue shades darker. Make-up to be worn in the evening is best applied under the type of lighting normally used at night, usually either electric filament lamps or warm white fluorescent lamps.

Preparation of the trolley for make-up

The trolley and required materials should be prepared prior to the arrival of the client. Preparation of the following items should be made at the same time but these should be kept in a UV cabinet until required.
1. Spatulas and make-up pallette.
2. Orange sticks and cotton buds.
3. Make-up brushes (see Fig. 14.2).
4. Make-up sponges or wedges.

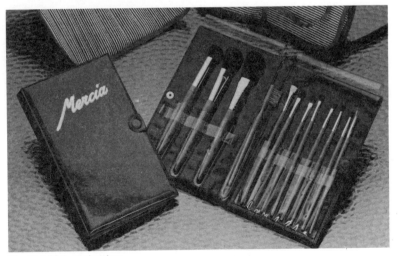

Fig. 14.2 Make-up brushes

The equipment required on the trolley is as follows:
1. Client record card.
2. Tissues.
3. Damp cotton wool pads.

4. Dry cotton wool pads.
5. Sterilising fluid (for the insertion of spatulas).
6. Headband.
7. Towels.
8. Mirror .
9. Choice of cleansers, e.g. liquid and cream.
10. Choice of toners, e.g. bracer and toner.
11. Choice of moisturisers, e.g. liquid and cream.
12. Green corrective cream and concealer sticks.
13. Selection of foundations.
14. Blushers/highlighters/shaders.
15. Translucent powder.
16. Eye shadows/mascara/eyeliner.
17. Lipstick/lip gloss.
18. Glitter.
19. False lashes.   } for evening make-up
20. Shimmering eye and face powder

Preparation of the client

1. Seat the client comfortably in an upright or a reclining position ensuring that her head and neck are well supported.
2. Ask the client to remove any ear-rings or necklaces, and keep these in a safe place.
3. Place a clean gown or towel around the client's shoulders ensuring that the clothing is adequately covered. Gently ease the client's hair back off the face and place a clean headband around the hairline in order to keep the hair off the face while treatment is being carried out.
4. Consult the client's record card and discuss her requirements with her. A client make-up chart (see Fig. 14.3) may then be completed.

Order of application of make-up

1. Cleansers, toners and moisturisers (see Chapter 7).
2. Blemish concealers.
3. Foundation (to suit skin type).
4. Cream products, if being used, are applied at this stage, e.g. cream blusher, highlighter, shader and cream eye shadow.
5. Translucent powder to set the creams.
6 Powder products, if being used, are applied at this stage, e.g. shaders, highlighters, blushers and eye shadows.
Note: Cream products are always applied on top of cream since they are of the same consistency and will blend easily with the foundation. Powder products are always applied after the application of translu-

Make-up chart

Name of client...

Date.............................

Face shape...
Spectacles/contact lenses ....
Occasion ....
Areas for corrective make-up.......................

Cosmetics to be applied
                 Type   *Colour*
Foundation ....
Blusher..
Shaders ....
Highlighters ....
Eye make-up ....
                  ....
Lip make-up ....

Fig. 14.3 Make-up chart

cent powder as they blend more easily with the powder than they would if put directly on to the foundation.

7. Mascara and eyeliner.
8. Lipstick and lip gloss.

On completion of the make-up the face should be checked to ensure that the application is even. It may be necessary to re-touch with powder blushers and to re-brush the eyebrows. If the client approves of the make-up, remove the headband and tidy the client's hair. A record card (see Fig. 14.4) should then be completed. Brushes, spatulas, etc. should be washed and replaced in the UV cabinet, and the area tidied ready for the next client.

Cosmetic Make-up Record Card

Name of client...

Address...

....

....

Tel. no ....

Face shape..

Skin type ....

Medical factors which may affect treatment
Allergies ....
Skin abnormalities......................................
Any health problems ....
Drugs being taken......................................
Spectacles/contact lenses ....

Date	Treatment	Remarks	Cosmetician

Fig. 14.4 Record card

The make-up of black skin

Careful examination is required during the skin analysis of black skin since skin lesions are less easily visible than on lighter skins. Erythema (redness of the skin) appears only as purple patches which are often difficult to detect. The sebaceous glands and their ducts are usually large and follicles may be filled with sebum or contain small cysts which are obvious only to the touch. The epidermis is thicker and desquamation greater than in white skin and may result in a slight grey cast on the skin. Removal of the dead cells from the skin surface thus helps to improve the colour of the skin, and the cleansing process may be quite vigorous.

Black skin may appear shiny without necessarily being greasy, partly due to lack of vellus hair on the face. Matt make-up products are thus often preferable. If pigmentation of the skin is patchy, corrective make-up may be necessary to even out the colour before the foundation is applied.

On unblemished skin, a tinted gel foundation is sufficient as this has little covering power. Otherwise a non-greasy foundation of a golden brown or slightly orange shade may be used.

Blusher is important as the prominent cheek bones are often an attractive feature and require highlighting. Non-greasy blushers or gels in shades of deep red, orange red, vivid pink or wine will add suitable colour to the cheeks. In general, highlighters are more suitable for contouring than shaders which often tend to be invisible on dark skin. The appearance of a broad flat nose may be improved by the application of highlighter down the middle length of the nose or to correct wide nostrils a dark chestnut shadow may be applied along each side.

Translucent powders and powders prepared for use on white skin are unsuitable for dark skin. Those designed specially for black skin are prepared without the addition of titanium dioxide or zinc oxide which would make the powder too white and give a chalky appearance and a sallow colour. Suitable powders should have the same colour as the foundation. Fine powders are the most satisfactory as these have greater adherence.

Pressed powders are the most suitable type of eye shadow, using deep-coloured matt shadows of emerald green, orange brown or golden beige for day wear and pearlised shadows of sapphire blue, almond green or gold for evening wear. Light colours are usually much less effective. Kohl pencils or eyeliners may be used to accentuate the eyes.

The lips may be thick and wide and of similar colour to the skin. Light-coloured and glossy lipsticks should therefore be avoided. Dark colours will make the lips appear smaller: dark red, brick red, vivid pink or purple lipsticks with good staying power are most suitable.

No attempt should be made to impose European style make-up and detailed consultation with the client is of prime importance.

Questions

1. Explain why a day make-up often proves more difficult to carry out than an evening make-up.
2. Why does lighting play an important part when selecting colours for evening make-up?
3. Explain what is meant by 'a total look' and give an example.
4. Name three cosmetics which would be used specifically for evening make-up only and explain the reason for their use.
5. How would you choose a suitable day make-up for a black skin, particularly with regard to the colours selected?

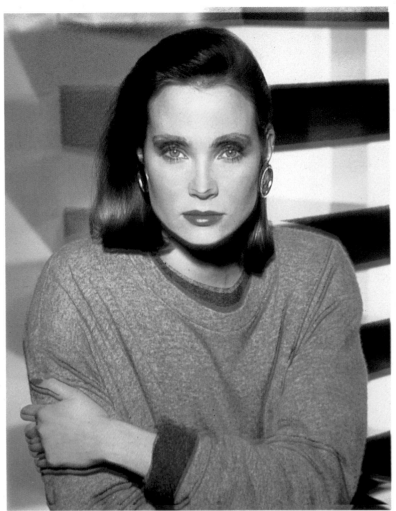

Bright version of day make-up using Estee Lauder's new Blueprints and Urbane Make-up Collection for Spring "88

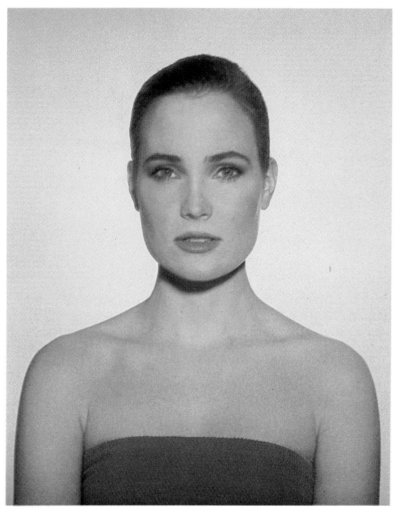

A more muted softer make-up for the evening using Estee Lauder's Signature range.

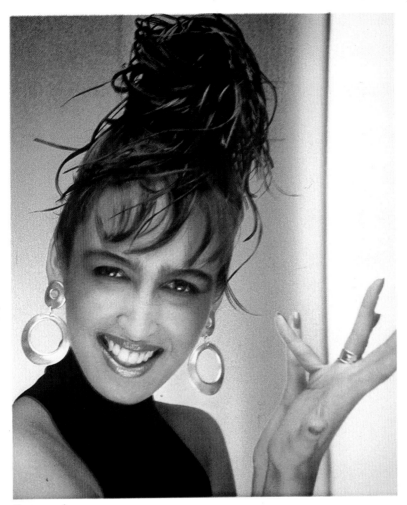

Fantasy make-up

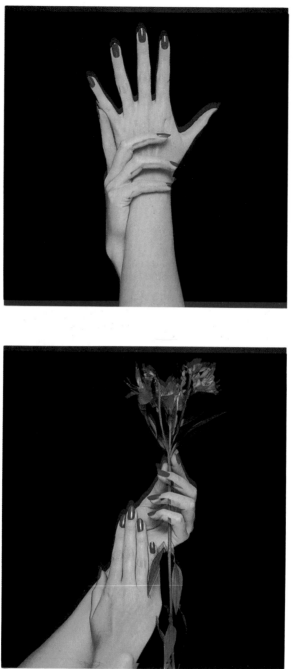

Completed manicure

Chapter 15

False eyelashes

False eyelashes can be an aid to fashion trends and are particularly useful for photographic, evening and fantasy make-ups. Short straight lashes can be enhanced to appear long and curled. It is not usual to use excessively thick false lashes other than for photographic work. Fine lashes have a much more natural appearance since they blend easily with the client's own lashes. Eyelash curlers may be used to curl false lashes, either once they are in place or before applying them to the eyelids.

There are two basic types of false eyelashes:
1. *strip lashes or complete sets of lashes*;
2. *semi-permanent lashes or individual eyelashes.*

Strip lashes

These are purchased in pairs forming a complete set of lashes. They are made from human hair or nylon fibres attached to a very fine backing strip. This may be either a self-adhesive strip or may require the application of a special eyelash adhesive which is normally supplied with the lashes. No other type of adhesive should be used. Lashes are available in various lengths and may be trimmed according to requirements, though care should be taken to ensure that their natural appearance is not lost. Individual lashes, especially those closest to the nose, may be shortened to follow the line of the client's own lashes. Strip lashes also vary in thickness from fine to heavy and colours range from black to light brown.

Application of strip lashes

False eyelashes are usually applied before carrying out the eye make-up. It may be thought necessary to test the adhesive on the client's skin prior to application, in order to detect any contra-indication. This is rare but may occur on skins which are particularly sensitive. The test should be carried out in the same way as for eyelash tints.

Procedure
1. Prepare the trolley with strip lashes, adhesive, sterilised tweezers and eyelash curlers.
2. Ensure that your hands are scrupulously clean.

3. Make sure that the client is in a comfortable position.
4. In consultation with the client and taking into account the eye and face shape, select the appropriate lashes ensuring that those chosen give a natural effect and that the client herself will feel comfortable while wearing them.
5. Using sterile tweezers, take one strip and apply adhesive from the tube directly on to the backing strip.
6. Ask the client to close her eyes and, with the lashes still in the tweezers, carefully position them over her own lashes (see Fig. 15.1). Ensure that they are placed as close to the roots as possible and then gently press into place along the eyelid. (Keep the adhesive away from the natural lashes otherwise they may stick together.)

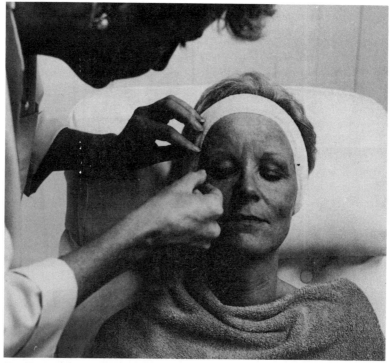

Fig. 15.1 Application of false eyelashes

7. Apply a strip lash to the other eye in the same way.
8. Check that both sets of lashes are correctly positioned and that they match. If there is any discrepancy, carefully ease them into position.
9. Allow the adhesive to set for approximately 3 minutes before continuing the make-up.
10. The lashes may be curled by using eyelash curlers to give a more luxuriant appearance. Eyelash curlers (see Fig. 1.1) are scissor-like

implements with rubber-covered blades, curved to correspond to the curve of the eyelid. The open blades are placed over the lashes of the half-closed eyes and gently squeezed to give lift to the lashes. Extreme care must be taken, however, to avoid trapping the skin of the eyelids when using curlers. A thin coat of mascara applied before the use of the curlers will help to protect the lashes during curling.

Removal of strip lashes

To remove strip lashes, gently peel them off from the outer to inner corner of the eye. A moistened cotton wool pad may be gently wiped over the closed eyelids and lashes to remove any traces of adhesive.

Care of strip lashes and advice to the client

Strip lashes may be used more than once and the client will require advice on treatment and storage. After removal from the eyelids, peel the adhesive from the backing strip and then place the lashes in warm water for a few minutes to remove any remaining adhesive. On removal from the water, place the lashes on a clean tissue, gently pat dry, and then roll them over a pencil to retain their curled shape. Slide the lashes off the pencil and reshape them in the box provided.

Semi-permanent or individual lashes

Individual lashes give a far more natural effect than strip lashes. They also take much longer to apply since they are used singly, each single unit comprising approximately three lashes. They are normally obtainable in boxes of 60 and can be purchased in different lengths. The colour range is from black to brown.

They may remain in position for about six weeks but often become detached and need replacing before that time due to normal wear and tear. Some clients may have a sensitivity to artificial lashes or the adhesive and may not be able to wear them. However, individual lashes are often preferred because they are lighter than strip lashes and adhere to the natural lashes rather than to the skin. Extra-strong adhesive is needed to attach these lashes in order to obtain a firm hold. Only special eyelash adhesive should be used as no other adhesive would be safe or suitable.

Application of individual lashes

It is usual to apply false eyelashes before carrying out the eye make-up. Some clients may be sensitive to the strong adhesive used for this type of lash. It may thus be necessary to test the skin for allergy at least 24 hours prior to the intended time of application, by applying a small amount of adhesive to the skin in the fold of the elbow.

Procedure

1. Prepare the trolley with lashes, adhesive, sterilised tweezers and a sterilised dish or palette.
2. Ensure your hands are scrupulously clean.
3. Prepare the client ensuring that she is in a comfortable position.
4. Consult the client to determine the effect, colour and length of lashes required, always taking into account the eye and face shape before the final selection.
5. Squeeze a small amount of adhesive into a small sterilised dish or on to a sterilised palette.
6. Ask the client to keep her eyes open and to tilt her head downwards very slightly, so partially lowering the eyelids.
7. Working from behind the client, select a lash using sterile tweezers, and dip the root end into the adhesive.
8. Work from the inner corner to the outer corner of the top lid. Using a stroking movement, gently glide the root over the client's own lashes and then carefully ease it back up the lashes, bringing it to rest at the root of the natural lashes as near to the lid as possible. Follow the same procedure across the eyelid, pausing after each application to enable adhesion to take place.
9. On completion, check the application before proceeding to the other eye.
10. When both upper lids are completed, check that they match before proceeding to the lower lashes.
11. If watering of the eyes occurs, stop the application and allow the client to sit up until it ceases.
12. Application to the lower lashes is usually done from the front, following the same procedure as that for the upper lashes.

Removal of individual lashes

Individual lashes are removed by use of an adhesive solvent. Using a cotton wool tipped orange stick, apply a little solvent to the base of the eyelash while the client's eyes are closed. Pause for a second or two and then draw the tip gently down the lash to remove it. Treat all the false lashes in the same manner. If some appear stubborn, they may need another application of solvent to remove them. This type of lash is normally discarded after use.

Precautions

1. Use sterilised materials at all times.
2. Do not work erratically around the eyes.
3. Do not allow the adhesive to come into contact with the eyes.
4. Avoid the use of excess adhesive which may cause adhesion of the top and bottom lashes.

5. Avoid using very long lashes on clients who wear spectacles since they may brush the lenses and cause discomfort.

Contra-indications to the use of false lashes

1. Possible reaction to the adhesive.
2. Eye disorders, e.g. styes, blepharitis and conjunctivitis.
3. Inflammation or swelling of the tissues in the area of the eyes.

Questions

1. Give three reasons why clients may wish to wear false eyelashes.
2. What are the advantages of using semi-permanent or individual lashes in preference to strip lashes?
3. What factors would affect the choice of thickness and length of false lashes?
4. What advice would you give to a client requesting false lashes if the client:
   (a) were known to have a sensitive skin;
   (b) had slight inflammation of one eyelid;
   (c) wears spectacles?
5. At what stage of make-up are false eyelashes normally applied?

Chemicals for cosmetic make-up

Alcohol (ethanol)	Surgical spirit. Used for disinfection of tools. Suspending agent for pigment in liquid foundations, lipstick and mascara. Used in toners as an astringent.
Almond oil	Vegetable oil. Used in oil phase of cold cream, cleansing cream and night creams. Also in warm oil face masks and in calamine face packs for sensitive dry skin.
Aluminium chlorohydrate	Astringent used in toners and antiperspirants.
Aluminium hydroxide	Used to prepare insoluble coloured lakes from soluble coal-tar dyes.
Aluminium silicate	Clay. *See* bentonite, fuller's earth and kaolin.
Aluminium stearate	Gelling agent used in gel foundations to produce a jelly-like consistency.
Antimony sulphide	Kohl. Used in eyeliner pencils.
Beeswax	Used with borax as an emulsifying agent for cleansing creams. Wax base of lipsticks, eye liner and eyebrow pencils. Wax face masks.
Bentonite	Grey-white clay obtained from volcanic ash. Used in clay-based face packs. Thickens and suspends pigments in liquid foundations and lip gloss.
Bismuth oxychloride	Pearliser obtained from fish scales or made synthetically. Added to eye shadows and lipstick.
Calamine	Pale pink powder of zinc carbonate. Mixed with water or rose-water in face packs for sensitive skins.
Calcium thioglycollate	Used in chemical depilatory creams.
Candelilla wax	Yellow-brown hard wax obtained from a plant and used in wax base of lipstick.
Carnauba wax	Hard wax obtained from surface of palm leaves used as hardener in lipstick, eyeline pencil, and cake foundations. Water-repellant in mascara.

Castor oil	Vegetable oil used in lipstick and liquid mascara.
Ceresin (purified ozokerite)	Micro-crystalline earth wax used in emulsions to reduce greasiness by absorbing oils. Added to foundation cream, lipstick and eye shadow.
Cetrimide	Used in antiseptic creams and as liquid for sterilising tools.
Cetyl alcohol	White waxy solid. Emulsifying agent for cleansing creams. Also in eyeliner and eyebrow pencils.
Chalk (precipitated)	Used in translucent powders to produce a velvety appearance (bloom).
Chromium oxide	Gives green colour to green corrective creams and foundations for blemish covering.
Eosin (bromo-acid dye)	Staining colour for lipstick. Potential sensitiser.
Fuller's earth	Hydrous aluminium silicate. Grey powder used in clay face packs.
Gelatin	Used in gel peel-off face masks.
Glycerol (glycerine)	Humectant and emollient. Added to astringent lotions and moisturising creams.
Gum acacia	Gum used in gel face masks.
Gum tragacanth	Gum used in gel face masks, gel foundations and liquid lipstick.
Hexaclorophene	Antiseptic added to toners and medicated foundations.
Hydrogen peroxide	Oxidising agent used with eyebrow and eyelash tints. Added to clay packs to lighten skin.
Iron oxide	Inorganic pigment (umber, sienna and ochre) used in foundations, lipstick and eye shadow.
Isopropyl myristate	Oily liquid used to reduce greasiness of cream products
Kaolin (China clay)	Hydrous aluminium silicate. White powder used in clay packs. Also in face powder, cream highlighters, all-in-one and cake foundations.
Lanolin	Similar to sebum but obtained from sheep's wool. Added as emollient to many products. Potential sensitiser.
Magnesium carbonate	White powder. Mild astringent used in clay packs.
Magnesium silicate	*See* talc.
Magnesium stearate	Used in translucent powder to increase ad-

	hesion. Also as binding agent in cake make-up.
Menthol	Obtained from oil of peppermint. Astringent in toners.
Methyl cellulose	Thickener for liquid lipstick, eyeliner and mascara. Gelling agent in gel eye shadow.
Mineral oil	Petroleum product used in most cosmetic creams, lipstick, cake and pencil eyeliner, eyebrow pencil, cake foundation and mascara.
Olive oil	Vegetable oil used in warm oil face masks. Ingredient of superfatted soap.
Orange flower water	Perfumed water used as mild astringent in skin tonics and fresheners.
Ozokerite	Hard white micro-crystalline earth wax used to partially replace mineral oil in cream products to reduce greasiness.
Paraffin wax	Petroleum product used as thickener in creams, also in wax face masks and depilatory wax.
Petroleum jelly	Petroleum product used in wax face masks, in lipstick, eyeline pencils and many cosmetic creams. Also to protect surrounding skin in eyelash and eyebrow tinting.
Polyvinyl pyrrolidone	Plastic resin used to thicken liquid products such as eyeliner and mascara. Also in gel face masks.
Rose water	Perfumed water used as mild astringent in skin tonics and fresheners. Also to mix clay packs for sensitive or dry skin.
Silicone oils	Synthetic oil added to lipstick to improve spreading properties.
Sodium hypochlorite	Sterilising fluid for tools.
Sorbitol	Humectant added to moisturising creams.
Spermaceti wax	White wax obtained from whales. Used in liquifying cleansing creams.
Stearic acid	White waxy solid used in moisturising creams.
Sulphonated castor oil	Used in non-greasy cleansing creams. Also to mix calamine face packs for very dry skin.
Sulphur	Yellow powder used in clay-based face packs for acnefied skins.
Talc (magnesium silicate)	Fine powder used in face powder, all-in-one foundations and cake cosmetics.
Titanium dioxide	Intensely white powder used to make products such as foundations and concealer cosmetics more opaque and improve their

	covering power. Added to lipstick dyes to give pastel shades.
Toluenediamine	Oxidation dye used for eyebrow and eyelash tinting. Potential sensitiser.
Triethanolamine lauryl sulphate	A soapless detergent used in non-greasy cleansers.
Triethanolamine stearate	A mild soap used in cream mascara and cake mascara.
Witch hazel	Astringent obtained from leaves and twigs of shrub (Hamamelis virginiana). Used in toners and to mix clay-based packs for greasy skin.
Zinc oxide	Intensely white slightly astringent powder used in face powder and foundations to make them more opaque.

Multiple choice questions for cosmetic make-up

In each of the following questions, choose the most suitable answer from the four alternatives given.

1. The muscle which raises the eyebrows and wrinkles the forehead is the
   (a) temporalis
   (b) corrugator supercilii
   (c) pyramidalis
   (d) frontalis

2. The number of bones in the cranium is
   (a) 7
   (b) 8
   (c) 14
   (d) 22

3. The only movable bone of the skull is the
   (a) mandible
   (b) maxilla
   (c) zygomatic
   (d) sphenoid

4. Crow's feet are found
   (a) on the neck
   (b) at the corners of the mouth
   (c) around the eyes
   (d) at the base of the nose

5. The horny layer of the epidermis is also known as the
   (a) stratum germinativum
   (b) stratum granulosum
   (c) stratum lucidum
   (d) stratum corneum

6. The two types of fibres contained in the dermis are called
   (a) collagen and keratin
   (b) elastic fibres and keratin
   (c) collagen and elastic fibres
   (d) elastic fibres and fibroblasts

7. Contraction of the arrector pili muscle results from
   (a) stimulation by a motor nerve
   (b) stimulation by a sensory nerve
   (c) the action of elastic fibres in the dermis
   (d) the movement of the hair follicle

8. Ageing of the skin may be due to
   (a) loss of elasticity of collagen
   (b) degeneration of elastic fibres
   (c) excess subcutaneous fat
   (d) over-activity of the sebaceous glands

9. The tan produced by UVA is
   (a) delayed and long-lasting
   (b) delayed and temporary
   (c) immediate and temporary
   (d) immediate and long-lasting

10. A blackhead is also called a
    (a) pustule
    (b) macule
    (c) comedo
    (d) papule

11. Which one of the following is a macule?
    (a) a whitehead
    (b) a freckle
    (c) a mole
    (d) a verruca

12. A keloid is
    (a) an overgrown scar
    (b) a type of protein
    (c) a pigment in the skin
    (d) a bone in the skull

13. Which one of the following is caused by a bacterial infection?
    (a) impetigo
    (b) psoriasis
    (c) ringworm
    (d) cold sore

14. The term 'erythema' refers to
    (a) heat treatment of the skin
    (b) treatment by ultra-violet rays
    (c) tanning of the skin
    (d) redness of the skin

15. The most suitable astringent for a greasy skin is
    (a) witch hazel
    (b) cetrimide
    (c) purified water
    (d) rose water

16. The most suitable astringent for a dry skin is
    (a) witch hazel
    (b) alcohol
    (c) cetrimide
    (d) rose water

17. The main function of a moisturiser is to
    (a) prevent acne
    (b) maintain the water content of the skin
    (c) remove make-up
    (d) exclude moisture from the skin

18. Toning is carried out after cleansing to
    (a) remove any trace of grease
    (b) relax the client
    (c) put oil back into the skin
    (d) dry up any skin blemishes

19. A fuller's earth face pack is most suitable for
    (a) dry skin
    (b) greasy skin
    (c) skin with open pores
    (d) acnefied skin

20. A calamine face pack is most suitable for
    (a) dry skin
    (b) greasy skin
    (c) skin with open pores
    (d) acnefied skin

21. Automatic tweezers are used to
    (a) remove bulk from the eyebrow
    (b) achieve the final eyebrow shape
    (c) remove lashes
    (d) curl eyelashes

22. Eyebrow shaping is contra-indicated if
    (a) the brows are very bushy
    (b) the client has a stye
    (c) the brows have been tinted
    (d) the client is rather elderly

23. Which of the following should be applied around the eye before carrying out an eyelash tint?
    (a) an antiseptic
    (b) a toner
    (c) petroleum jelly
    (d) a moisturiser

24. An eyelash tint should be mixed with
    (a) water
    (b) surgical spirit
    (c) 10 volume hydrogen peroxide
    (d) 20 volume hydrogen peroxide

25. Irritation occurring after using eyelash tint in a skin test may be relieved by applying
    (a) calamine
    (b) camomile
    (c) collodion
    (d) cleansing cream

26. If tint accidentally enters a client's eye, the cosmetician should
    (a) panic and send for medical assistance
    (b) leave the client and seek help from colleagues
    (c) immediately flush out the eye with water
    (d) remove the tint and flush out the eye with water

27. Red lipstick viewed under a pure blue light would appear
    (a) red
    (b) blue
    (c) purple
    (d) black

28. Concealer stick is used to
    (a) mask any redness of the skin
    (b) cover a cold sore
    (c) mask blemishes
    (d) cover a cut or abrasion

29. Foundations should be applied with
    (a) dry cotton wool
    (b) a damp sponge
    (c) a brush
    (d) a moist tissue

30. Green corrective cream is used to
    (a) enhance blue eye shadow
    (b) mask a ruddy complexion
    (c) complement a pale foundation
    (d) conceal dark circles

31. Powder blusher should be used
    (a) on top of the foundation
    (b) on top of cream products only
    (c) after the application of translucent powder
    (d) only on greasy skins

32. To correct the appearance of a long nose
    (a) shade the sides of the nose
    (b) highlight the tip of the nose
    (c) shade the tip of the nose
    (d) highlight the cheeks

33. Translucent powder is used
    (a) to set cream products
    (b) as a foundation
    (c) to conceal blemishes
    (d) to tone down high colouring

34. After use on a client, eyeliner pencils should be
    (a) placed in a bowl of disinfectant
    (b) discarded immediately
    (c) re-sharpened and placed in a UV cabinet
    (d) wiped with surgical spirit

35. Which one of the following substances is used as a pearliser in eye shadows?
    (a) titanium dioxide
    (b) bismuth oxychloride
    (c) ozokerite wax
    (d) iron oxide

36. The term 'an asymmetrical mouth' means that
    (a) the top and bottom lips are both the same shape
    (b) the top lip is larger than the bottom lip
    (c) the bottom lip is larger than the upper lip
    (d) one side of the top lip is narrower than the other

37. Which of the following lipstick ingredients is a known sensitiser?
    (a) eosin dye
    (b) mineral oil
    (c) ceresin
    (d) carnauba wax

38. A good lipstick should always
    (a) stain the lips
    (b) dry out any moisture present
    (c) fade slightly after application
    (d) be non-toxic

39. False eyelashes are contra-indicated if the client
    (a) wears glasses
    (b) uses contact lenses
    (c) is allergic to the adhesive
    (d) already has long lashes

40. Individual (semi-permanent) lashes are removed
    (a) each evening
    (b) by plucking
    (c) by use of a solvent
    (d) by steaming the face

Answers to multiple choice questions in cosmetic make-up

Question:	1	2	3	4	5	6	7	8	9	10
Answer:	(d)	(b)	(a)	(c)	(d)	(c)	(a)	(b)	(c)	(c)

Question:	11	12	13	14	15	16	17	18	19	20
Answer:	(b)	(a)	(a)	(d)	(a)	(d)	(b)	(a)	(b)	(a)

Question:	21	22	23	24	25	26	27	28	29	30
Answer:	(a)	(b)	(c)	(c)	(a)	(d)	(d)	(c)	(b)	(b)

Question:	31	32	33	34	35	36	37	38	39	40
Answer:	(c)	(c)	(a)	(c)	(b)	(d)	(a)	(d)	(c)	(c)

Part 3
Manicure

Chapter 16

The nails

Nails are appendages of the skin consisting of tough keratin plates designed to protect the ends of the fingers. They facilitate the picking up of small objects and are also useful as tools for scratching. They grow from the germinating layer of the epidermis in a similar way to the growth of hair.

The structure of nails

A section through the end of a finger showing the relationship of the nail to its surrounding structures is shown in Fig. 16.1.

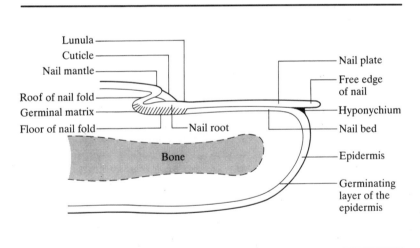

Fig. 16.1 Section through the end of a finger

The nail plate

The main body of the nail is called the *nail plate*. About one-fifth of the plate, *the nail root*, lies under the *nail fold* at the base of the nail. The *free edge* of the nail plate projects beyond the end of the digits (the fingers and thumbs) as a white or yellowish margin which is detached from the skin. The plate itself is a hard translucent structure made from a particularly compact form of protein keratin, which is sometimes termed *onychin* to distinguish it from other types of keratin. In normal health the plates curve in two directions, transversely from side to side across the nail and longitudinally from the base of the nail to the free edge.

The water content of the nail plate affects the relative pliability or brittleness of the nail. The normal water content is about 12 per cent for nails in a good pliable condition. At lower percentages the nails become brittle and tend to split or flake. Nails contain a very low percentage of fat, normally only 0.15–0.75 per cent by weight. The chief mineral element is calcium, but it is present only as 0.1 per cent so is considered to have little effect on the hardness of nails. There are no blood vessels or nerves in the nail plate.

The nail matrix

The nail grows from the *germinal matrix* which forms the floor of the nail fold, and also extends a short way forwards to be visible through the nail plate as the white area at the base of the nail known as the *lunula* or half moon. The matrix itself consists of cells of germinating layer and prickle cell layer of the epidermis, the granular layer being absent from all parts of the matrix. A few melanocytes are usually present but their effect is rarely noticeable except in some negroid people who develop dark longitudinal lines along the nail plate.

The nail bed

Immediately under the nail plate is the *nail bed*. The two structures are firmly attached to each other except at the tip of the fingers where the nail plate separates to form the free edge of the nail. The epidermal tissue under the nail at this point of separation is called the *hyponychium*. The nail bed itself consists of a few layers of living epidermal tissue and the underlying dermis. At the junction between the dermis and epidermis in the nail bed, instead of the dermal papillae of normal skin, the dermis is arranged in a series of grooves and ridges running the length of the nail. The folds fit into a similar series of ridges and grooves in the epidermis and give firm adhesion of the nail plate to the nail bed. The dermis below the nail plate is well supplied with blood capillaries which are visible through the nail plate giving the nails their normal pink colour. The nail bed also contains many sensory nerve endings, hence the great sensitivity to pain if a nail plate is lost.

The cuticle

The cuticle (see Fig. 16.2) is an extension of the horny layer of the epidermis from the nail fold (this part of the nail fold is sometimes referred to as the *nail mantle*) on to the nail plate. The function of the cuticle is to protect the germinal matrix by making a water-tight joint so preventing the entry of bacteria and other micro-organisms into the area under the nail fold. The *eponychium* lies behind the cuticle and is also an extension of the horny layer of the epidermis on to the nail plate. It arises from the roof of the nail fold and is often considered to be part of the cuticle.

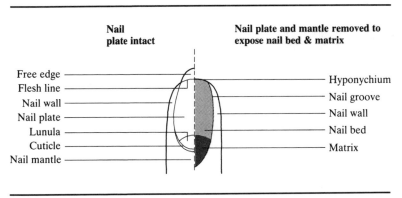

Fig. 16.2 Last joint of a finger to show parts of a nail

The growth of nails

Nails develop in the embryo by the folding of the epidermis to form the nail fold which covers the germinal matrix of the nail. The fold appears as a thickened area on each finger at about the third month of development, and nail formation is completed at about the fifth month when they reach the tips of the fingers.

Growth of nails takes place by cell division in the matrix. Older cells are pushed forward as new ones are produced, and gradually they harden and die as their nuclei are destroyed and keratinisation takes place. The cells become firmly stacked together, held by a strong *cementing material* which is secreted by the cells themselves into the spaces between them, resulting in their adhesion to form the tough nail plate. The nail bed is also thought to be involved in the formation of the nail plate. New cells produced in the germinating layer of the nail bed are pushed forwards by the movement of the upper nail plate and become attached to it, so forming the lower part of the plate. In fact the nail plate is considered to consist of three layers closely bonded together, each developing from a different part of the matrix or from the nail bed. (This explains why the nail plate often separates and splits off in layers if the nails are brittle.) The direction of growth of the nail plate is shown in Fig. 16.3.

As the nail grows it moves along furrows or *nail grooves* at the sides of the nail. The grooves are protected by folds of skin, the *nail walls*, which

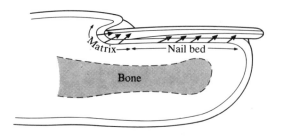

Fig. 16.3 Direction of growth of a nail plate

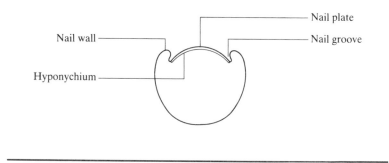

Fig. 16.4 Surface view of end of finger showing the nail grooves

slightly overlap the nail plate (see Fig. 16.4). The nail walls and the nail fold at the base of the nail together form the *perionychium*.

Unlike hair which has a cyclic growth pattern, the growth of nails is continuous throughout life. The rate of growth varies from person to person but is normally about 3–5 mm per month, being faster in youth than in old age. It takes about 3 months for cells to travel from the lunula to the tip of the nail, and 4–5 months for re-growth if a nail is completely lost. More rapid growth is noted in the longer fingers than the shorter, and in right-hand nails rather than left-hand nails. During illness growth is usually slowed, though in the case of psoriasis nail growth is faster due to an increased rate of cell division. The action of ultra-violet rays also speeds cell division, so nails grow faster in summer than in winter. Damage to a nail plate can only be repaired by the nail growing out, since the nail itself is a dead structure. This will only take place if the matrix remains undamaged.

The blood supply to the nails

Arterial blood is carried to the finger tips by the digital arteries (see Fig. 16.5). These branch many times to surround the bones of the fingers, and capillary networks from these branches give a rich blood supply to the germinal matrix, the nail bed and other structures around the nails. The growth of nails is dependant on nutrients and oxygen brought to the matrix by the blood. This enables cell division and keratinisation to take place during the formation of the nail plate. Nail deformities often occur due to poor circulation in these capillaries, the effect being increased if they are contracted in cold weather.

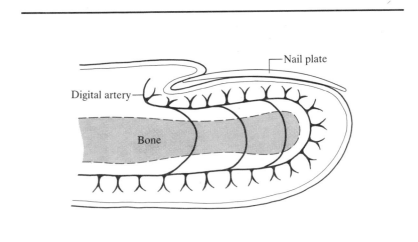

Fig. 16.5 Blood supply to a nail

The effect of age on the nails

The circulation of the blood in the nail bed and matrix becomes less efficient as ageing takes place, leading to a gradual slowing of nail growth. The effect may be increased by possible nutritional deficiency, especially lack of iron in the diet which decreases the blood supply. The nails tend to become thicker and therefore more opaque, so that the colour of the blood in the nail bed can no longer be clearly seen through the nail plate, and the nails thus become yellow or grey. Longitudinal ridges often become more pronounced and more numerous. The moisture-holding capacity of the nails is usually reduced, making them more fragile. They often then either split into layers at the free edge or develop longitudinal fissures.

Questions

1. What is meant by each of the following?
   (a) the hyponychium
   (b) the lunula
   (c) the perionychium
2. Describe the part played by the nail bed in the development and growth of nails.
3. Explain why the nails are normally pink, but in old age they may be yellow or grey.
4. What is the function of the following?
   (a) the nail grooves
   (b) the nail walls
   (c) the cuticle
5. From which layer of the skin does a nail grow?
   What factors affect nail growth?

Chapter 17

Nail and skin disorders affecting manicure

Before carrying out any treatment, the manicurist must examine the client's nails and note their condition. A healthy nail is smooth, shiny, pink and flexible, but many minor defects and some more serious disorders may result in changes in nail colour and structure, possibly affecting the type of manicure offered or being contra-indicative of manicure. The manicurist must thus be able to recognise common disorders and diseases of the nails so that a sound judgement about treatment may be made. If necessary, the client must be tactfully advised to seek medical attention.

Nail imperfections and diseases

Disorders and defects of the nail may arise from internal physiological conditions such as poor blood circulation, anaemia and psoriasis. Other conditions may be self-inflicted by misuse, accident or nervous habit. Diseases of the nails result from infection by micro-organisms such as ringworm fungus, yeasts and bacteria. Occasionally nails may be congenitally absent.

Defects of the nail plate

Brittle nails (fragilitas unguium)
Nails may be congenitally brittle, but more common reasons for brittleness are a low water content of the nail plate and a deficient blood supply to the matrix. Frequent use of detergents may lead to dehydration of the nail by constant removal of the protective oils. Poor circulation or iron deficiency anaemia may impair growth and lead to thinning of the nail plate. Water is more easily lost from a thin nail and brittleness may follow.

The eating of gelatin (table-jelly cubes) is sometimes recommended for the treatment of brittle nails but has no scientific foundation. Gelatin is a protein but is lacking in certain essential amino acids. During digestion all proteins are broken down into their individual amino acids and used for general body building and repair of tissues. Gelatin has no advantage over any other protein.

The use of cuticle cream massaged into the nail area at night, and avoidance of over-use of detergents or over-exposure to dry atmospheric conditions will be beneficial. The use of nail enamels is not contra-indicated since the film of enamel will delay water loss from the nail plate. Hard enamels containing nylon fibres may help to prevent nail breakage.

Eggshell nails

Thinning of the nail plate may result from defective circulation possibly due to ageing or anaemia. The nails bend easily and are often curved at the free edge (see Fig. 17.1) at which point they may break off. Unless kept short there is also a danger of separation of the nail from the nail bed (onycholysis) by leverage. The regular use of cuticle massage cream may improve circulation.

Furrows and ridges

Minor transverse furrows denote slight changes in growth rate of the nail, for example during a menstrual period. Numerous deeper furrows may appear as a result of dermatitis but are more usually caused by over-vigorous manicuring with frequent damage to the nail root.

A single transverse furrow or *Beau's line* (see Fig. 17.2), affecting all nails on both hands, may follow a serious illness such as measles, pneumonia or coronary thrombosis. The lines are due to a temporary interference with nail growth and appear several weeks after the illness when nail growth has returned to normal. The lines may take 3–4 months to grow out but no treatment is required.

Longitudinal ridges (see Fig. 17.3) are common even in good health, but tend to become more prominent in old age. They are also associated with rheumatoid arthritis when the ridging may be beaded. A single longitudinal groove may result from the nervous habit of picking at the cuticle area so damaging the nail root (see Fig. 17.12). Longitudinal ridging may be reduced by buffing the nails using a chamois leather buffing pad and a mild abrasive powder or pumice.

Hang nail (ag nail)

A hang nail is a small hard spike of nail growing in the nail groove alongside though separate from the main nail plate (see Fig. 17.4). It may result from injury to the nail root, biting the nails, dryness of the nail plate, or it may be congenital. If allowed to grow, the spike may become a nuisance by being pulled away from the skin at its base and possibly resulting in infection of the area. If slight inflammation occurs it should be treated with an antiseptic cream. Common warts may develop along the nail wall if the wart virus enters broken skin at the seat of the hang nail. The spike of hang nails should be cut with sharp-pointed sterilised scissors.

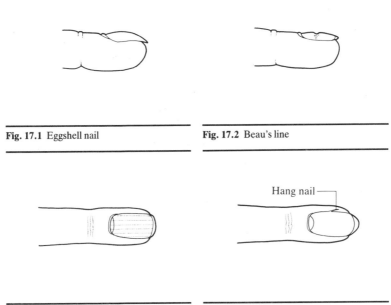

Fig. 17.1 Eggshell nail

Fig. 17.2 Beau's line

Fig. 17.3 Longitudinal ridges

Fig. 17.4 Hang nail

Hypertrophy and atrophy of nails
Hypertrophy or *onychauxis* refers to excessive thickening of the nails. It may be due to internal disorders or damage to the nail bed. The nails should be filed until razor thin.

Atrophy or *onychotrophia* means the wasting of the nails and is associated with diabetes and tuberculosis. The nails become gradually smaller and lack lustre. They should be treated gently and cut as smoothly and evenly as possible. Immersion of the hands in water and the use of detergents should be avoided.

Ingrowing nails
Ingrowing nails (onychocryptosis) are caused by cutting or filing the nail plate too low at the sides, which results in the nail growing into the flesh of the nail wall and causing inflammation. Toe nails are more frequently affected than finger nails.

Koilonychia (spoon-shaped nails)
In this condition the nails are typically spoon-shaped, being concave or depressed in the centre and raised at the outer edges (see Fig. 17.5); they are usually soft and thin. Middle-aged women often suffer from koilonychia since it is associated with iron deficiency anaemia. The cystine content of the nail keratin is low. Hairdressers may suffer from koilonychia

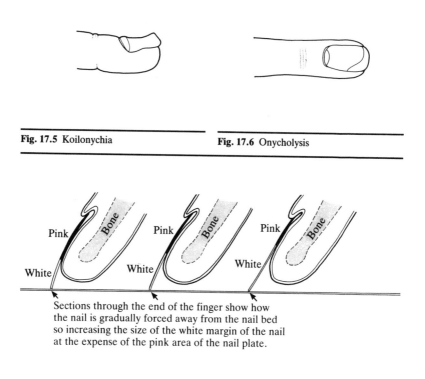

Fig. 17.5 Koilonychia

Fig. 17.6 Onycholysis

Sections through the end of the finger show how
the nail is gradually forced away from the nail bed
so increasing the size of the white margin of the nail
at the expense of the pink area of the nail plate.

Fig. 17.7 Nail forced from nail bed by leverage

due to frequent use of ammonium thioglycollate in perm lotion which
reduces the amount of the amino acid cystine in the nail plate. Medical
advice should be sought.

Onycholysis
Onycholysis is the premature separation of the nail from the nail bed at
the free edge of the nail or sometimes down one side of the nail plate (see
Fig. 17.6). It is visible as a white or yellowish extension of the nail
margin. The condition may be associated with psoriasis, dermatitis or
fungal infections. It may also be caused by an accidental trauma lifting
the nail away from the bed, or by over-vigorous cleaning of the underside
of the nail plate with a sharp instrument. The over-use of false nails may
cause onycholysis by interfering with the normal water balance of the
nails. The commonest cause, however, is pressure applied to the free
edge of the nail creating a lever action which forces the nail plate from
the bed (see Fig. 17.7). In this case the danger of onycholysis is greater
if the nail is narrow since the pressure is concentrated over a small area.

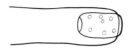

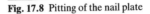

Fig. 17.8 Pitting of the nail plate

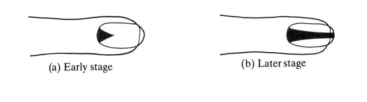

(a) Early stage   (b) Later stage

Fig. 17.9 Pterygium

There is a possibility of secondary infection if bacteria or fungi enter the enlarged space under the nail plate. Any manicure treatment, especially filing, must be carried out very gently. Shortening of the nails is advisable.

Onychoptosis
This involves the periodic shedding of nails and may be associated with other conditions such as alopecia universalis. If confined to one particular nail it may be due to permanent damage to the nail matrix.

Pitting of the nail plate
Thimble pitting (see Fig. 17.8) is usually secondary to another more serious condition. Deep pits are associated with psoriasis, shallow pits with alopecia areata, and coarser wider pits with dermatitis. Pitting is thought to be due to imperfect keratinisation resulting in small weak areas which are subsequently lost, leaving a hollow. Medical advice is necessary.

Psoriasis (effect on nails)
Psoriasis is a disorder due to abnormal keratinisation and may affect both the skin and the nails. Silvery scales may develop at the nail fold and under the free edge of the nail. The nail itself may become thickened due

to increased keratinisation in the nail bed. The growth of a horny layer in the nail bed is known as *onychophosis*. The lower part of the nail plate becomes a yellow-brown colour and is visible through the upper plate which is relatively unaffected. Thimble pitting of the surface of the nail may also occur. Psoriasis requires medical attention.

Pterygium unguium

This involves an overgrowth of the cuticle which becomes attached to the nail plate and grows forwards with it (see Fig. 17.9(a)). If left unchecked the pterygium can cover most of the nail, leaving only two small areas of the nail plate (see Fig. 17.9(b)). The condition may result from radiotherapy or be due to poor circulation to the matrix area. In extreme cases there may be loss of the nail. Oil manicure followed by cuticle clipping may be successful in the early stages. Otherwise medical advice should be sought.

Splitting of the nails

Onychorrhexis (see Fig. 17.10(a)) refers to longitudinal splitting of the nails. This often occurs along ridges, especially when they are deep. Ridging increases with age so that older people may suffer this defect, particularly if the nails are also thin and brittle. Careless filing during manicure may also cause splitting.

Onychoschizia or *lamellar dystrophy* (see Fig. 17.10(b)) refers to the splitting of the nail plate into layers. The nail splits horizontally through its thickness so that a flat portion breaks off at the free edge. The frequent immersion of the hands in water causes alternate swelling and then drying out of the nail with consequent splitting due to loss of adhesion between the cells of the nail plate. Flaking may also be caused by mechanical damage due to misuse of the nail. Protective gloves should be worn to avoid constant wetting of the hands; the nails should be kept short. Nail repair work may be carried out during manicure.

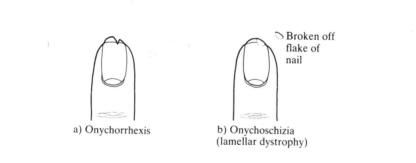

a) Onychorrhexis

b) Onychoschizia (lamellar dystrophy)

Broken off flake of nail

Fig. 17.10 Splitting of the nails

Self-inflicted damage to the nail area

These conditions result from nervous habits and would disappear if the habit could be overcome. Unfortunately, such habits are exceedingly difficult to break.

Nail biting (onychophagy)

Biting may result in distortion of the nail and may affect one particular nail or involve them all on both hands. The nails may be ragged and bitten down below the normal free edge (see Fig. 17.11). The habit usually starts in childhood and is exceptionally difficult to break. Treatment with unpleasant tasting substances is rarely successful. Frequent professional nail care and the use of coloured nail enamel may help, and they can often be improved one at a time. Cuticle massage may improve circulation and encourage growth. The bitten nails should be trimmed as smoothly and evenly as possible during manicure.

Cuticle biting

This may include biting the nail walls as well as the cuticle itself. The skin may be left ragged and may become infected if it is broken. Any protruding dead skin may be cut to tidy the area.

Picking of the nail or cuticle (onychotillomania)

The cuticle of the thumb is most usually attacked by the free edge of the nail on the first finger (the index finger) of the same hand. The cuticle and the nail root may be damaged, which may lead to infection of the nail fold resulting in inflammation and the formation of pus. Injury to the nail root may cause longitudinal grooving of the nail plate (see Fig. 17.12).

Discolouration of the nails

Nails may become discoloured by damage to the nail bed, fungal infection, or contact with various substances which stain the nail plate. Ringworm of the nail, a fungal infection, may cause it to be yellow, brown or black. Medical attention is required and no manicure service must be given. Hair dyes may stain the nail plate, tobacco stains (nicotine) cause yellowing, and some dark red nail enamels used without a base coat may also stain the nails.

Blue nails

Very pale or blue nails may indicate poor circulation in the nail bed, anaemia or possibly a heart condition. Frequent use of cuticle massage cream and massage of the fingers may stimulate the circulation.

Black or brown patches

Damage to the nail bed or to the matrix area may cause bleeding from capillaries in the dermis, leading to black or brown patches of dried

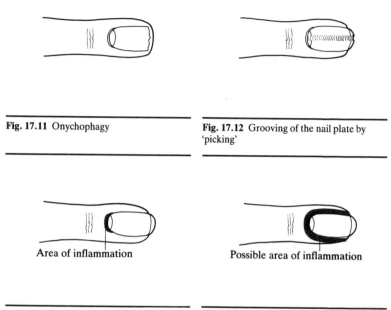

Fig. 17.11 Onychophagy

Fig. 17.12 Grooving of the nail plate by 'picking'

Area of inflammation

Possible area of inflammation

Fig. 17.13 Onychia

Fig. 17.14 Paronychia

blood under the nail plate. This happens, for instance, if the nail is trapped in a door or a heavy weight falls on to it. The patches grow out but the nail may be shed prematurely as the black area is detached from the nail bed.

Black streaks
These may grow along the length of the nail plate due to activity of melanocytes in the matrix. The condition most often occurs in dark-skinned races and is not considered to be of particular significance. Streaks may also arise after minor damage to the matrix in which case they will eventually grow out.

White spots (leuconychia puncta)
White spots on the nails may be caused by slight damage to the nail root or to the nail plate causing minor separation of the plate from the nail bed. The spots grow out and no special treatment is required.

Nail infections

Nail infections or onychoses are caused by micro–organisms such as bacteria and fungi.

Onychia
This is a recurring condition due to infection of the nail fold by a yeast-type fungus or by bacteria which gain entry through a damaged cuticle. Over-vigorous manicuring, cuticle picking, the over-use of detergents or excess treatment with cuticle remover may cause cuticle damage. Onychia often occurs in children who are habitual thumb-suckers, and in housewives and others whose hands are constantly exposed to moisture.

The nail fold and cuticle area may become inflamed (see Fig. 17.13). Pus is often formed and may be periodically expressed from beneath the nail fold. The inflammation tends to flare from time to time over a period of years. The condition can be exceedingly painful and difficult to eradicate. No manicure treatment should be given when inflammation is present. The hands should be kept dry where possible by using protective gloves. During periods when the condition clears, gentle manicure may be carried out but extreme care is required in dealing with the cuticle area.

Paronychia
Paronychia (see Fig. 17.14) refers to the inflammation of the skin round the nail. It may be caused by acute bacterial infection following any damage to the skin, to the use of unsterilised manicure tools or to a foreign body such as a splinter entering the skin. The inflamed area may be swollen and pus may form. The inflamed swelling is often termed a witlow or felon. The condition is painful but usually clears fairly quickly. No manicure treatment should be given until healing is complete.

Ringworm of the nail (onychomycosis)
The fungus (tinea unguium) causing ringworm of the nail attaches itself to the skin under the free edge of the nail (the hyponychium), and first attacks the nail bed and then the nail plate itself. The fungus secretes a digestive juice which splits keratin and uses it for nourishment. The first sign is a yellowish-brown discolouration at the free edge of the nail, which may later spread to the whole nail and also to other nails. The nail plate may become thickened (hypertrophied) and onycholysis may occur (see Fig. 17.15). No manicure treatment must be given if ringworm is suspected since it is contagious, and the client should be advised to seek medical help. Treatment usually consists of taking the drug griseofulvin orally and applying fungicidal creams to the area.

Dermatitis
Some substances, including some of those used in manicure, may cause irritation of the skin and nails. Some act as *primary irritants* and will affect any skin if contact time is sufficient. Primary irritants include the following:
1. Caustic alkalis, e.g. potassium hydroxide used in cuticle remover.
2. Enzyme detergents may damage the nail cuticle as well as causing

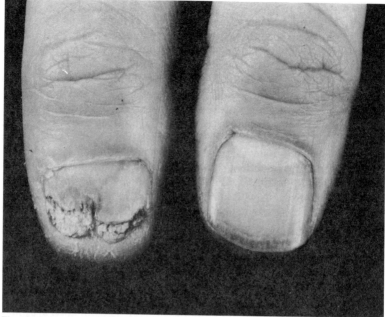

Fig. 17.15 Ringworm of the nail

dermatitis. Cuticle damage leaves the nail fold open to infection and onychia may follow.
3. Thioglycollates used in perm lotion and depillatory creams.
Other substances are known to be potential *sensitisers*, that is they may affect certain people who have become allergic to the substance by previous contact. Such substances may cause erythema with vesicles and papules and some swelling of the tissues. In cases of allergic reaction, the eruption is not confined to the area of contact but may in addition affect other areas of the skin. The nails may be affected by pitting, cross ridging and onycholysis. The nail bed may become dry and thickened. Substances applied to the nails, such as nail enamel, often cause allergic reaction in the more sensitive tissues around the eyes and on the neck rather than on the nails themselves, due to their contact with the skin of those areas. If a client has become allergic to any substance, complete avoidance of it is essential. Manicurists may, of course, be affected by allergy as well as clients.

Substances used in manicure which often cause sensitisation include:
1. The liquid monomer methyl methacrylate used for sculptured nails.
2. Formaldehyde resins used in nail enamels and nail hardeners.
3. Lanolin often used in nail enamel removers, hand creams, cuticle remover and cuticle massage creams.

Hypo-allergenic products are available from which well-known sensitisers have been omitted.

Skin conditions affecting manicure

Chilblains

Chilblains are irritant red swellings occurring on the fingers and are often troublesome in winter time. In severe cases the nail bed may be affected the nail plate may become detached. They are caused by poor circulation, a condition aggravated by cold. Manicure treatment should be avoided until all swelling disappears, then massage and finger exercises will help to improve circulation. The hands should always be kept warm by wearing gloves in cold weather.

Scabies

Infestation by itch mites (see Fig. 17.16) is known as scabies. The female mites burrow into the stratum corneum to lay eggs. The burrows can be seen as short, raised dark lines in the skin between the fingers or in the folds at the front of the wrists. The mites are easily passed from person to person by direct contact or on objects such as gowns and towels. No manicure treatment should be offered if scabies is suspected, and the client should be advised to seek medical attention.

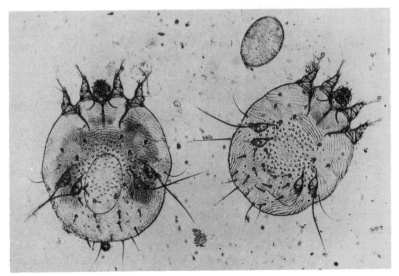

Fig. 17.16 Itch mite

Warts

Common warts often occur on the backs of the hands and, in association with hang nails, may also occur alongside the nails. They are caused by a virus infection of the epidermis resulting in a small area of abnormal keratinisation. The manicurist should avoid touching warts on clients' hands since they are contagious and clients should be advised to consult a doctor.

Questions

1. Describe the signs associated with the following:
   (a) bacterial infection of the skin around the nails;
   (b) infestation by itch mites;
   (c) ringworm of the nail;
   (d) damage to the nail bed.
2. What advice would you give to a client who:
   (a) complained of thin fragile nails;
   (b) developed badly ridged nails;
   (c) frequently bit her nails?
3. Describe the characteristics of a healthy nail.
   State two causes of discolouration of the nails.
4. What is meant by each of the following?
   (a) hang nails
   (b) onycholysis
   (c) a contagious disease
   (d) a witlow
5. Describe the ways in which a person may inflict damage on her own nails.

Chapter 18

Cosmetic preparations for the nails

Many of the products available for use on the nails are concerned with their adornment. These include nail enamels, buffing powders and nail whiteners. Associated with enamels are base and top coats, enamel removers, thinners and dryers. A few preparations, such as nail bleaches and strengtheners or hardeners, are used to improve nail condition. Products for use on the cuticles include cuticle remover and cuticle massage creams.

Nail enamel

Nail enamel is designed to enhance the appearance of the nails by the application of a tough glossy film which may either be coloured or clear.
   The film should possess the following characteristics:
1. It should adhere well to the nail plate and be thick enough, though sufficiently flexible to resist abrasion, chipping and peeling.
2. Good durability is required, including resistance to water, detergents and any other chemicals with which it may come into contact.
3. The colour should be fast to light and should stain neither the skin nor the nail plate.
4. It should be quick drying, forming an even film without brush marks.

The formulation of enamels

Nail enamel is basically a solution containing a *film former* (the solute) which carries the colour, dissolved in a *solvent* with suitable drying properties. On application to the nail, the solvent evaporates leaving a film of enamel on the nail plate. *Plasticisers* such as isopropyl myristate may be added to make the film more flexible, so reducing the possibility of the film cracking or chipping on the nail. To prepare an enamel which does not separate out on standing and therefore does not need shaking before use, bentonite clays are added. These enamels have a thick gel-like structure in the bottle but become liquid when brushed on to the nail.
   The film former is usually a mixture of nitrocellulose and a synthetic resin such as a formaldehyde resin or an acrylic resin. Used by itself, nitrocellulose has poor adhesion, is brittle and lacks gloss. The addition

of resins improves these qualities. The resins, however, are potential sensitisers and may cause an allergic reaction in certain people.

The solvent is a blend of volatile substances designed to give an enamel with a suitable rate of drying. If the solvent evaporates too quickly the enamel thickens on the nail and does not flow evenly, so that brush marks are left on the film. Rapid evaporation, taking latent heat from the nail, may also produce sufficient cooling to cause condensation of moisture from the air on to the nail surface, resulting in a cloudy film or 'bloom'. If less volatile solvents are used, the film may dry at an inconveniently slow rate. A solvent of suitable drying time usually consists of a carefully blended mixture of ethyl acetate, butyl acetate and toluene. Acetone is now rarely used as it is considered to be too drying to the nail and skin, and also increases the tendency to cloud since it evaporates rapidly.

The pigments used in nail enamels are usually synthetic dyes in the form of lakes, since these give bright colours. Iron oxide may be used to produce brown shades; titanium dioxide is added to give pastel shades and to make the colours more opaque or 'creamy'. Metallic powders made from gold leaf or aluminium are sometimes added.

Types of nail enamel

There are two types of enamel.
(a) *Cream enamel* which has a matt finish.
(b) *Crystalline enamel* which is pearlised by the addition of bismuth oxychloride (either synthetically produced or obtained from fish scales). This increases the amount of light reflected by the product and gives an iridescent finish.

Base coat

It is essential that a base coat is used before applying nail enamel. This gives added protection to the nail plates, masks any surface irregularities, prevents the staining of the nails by the enamel and helps to key the enamel to the nail plate.

The base coat differs in composition from enamel by containing:
1. A higher percentage of resins to improve adherence to the nail.
2. More volatile solvents to produce a quicker drying time.
3. Less plasticiser to give a harder coat.
4. Less pigment (or it may be pigment-free) to prevent staining of the nail.
5. A little hard wax such as carnauba wax which fills out any slight irregularities in the nail plate, so providing a smooth base of the enamel. Extra wax may be added in products intended for excessively ridged nails.

Top coat

This is applied only on top of cream enamels to give lustre and sheen, since pearlised enamels are already highly reflective. Top coat provides a colourless protective film to the enamel. Further applications of top coat may be made daily to give added protection to problem-type nails.
Top coat contains:

1. More nitrocellulose, more plasticiser and less resin than enamel to give a softer film, but with less adhesion since attachment to enamel is easier than to the nail plate.
2. More volatile solvents to give a quick drying time.

Nail enamel dryer

After the application of enamel, nail dryer may be sprayed on to the nails from an aerosol can to increase the speed of drying. The aerosol propellant evaporates quickly on the nails, carrying with it the solvent of the enamel. A transparent film of mineral oil is also deposited on the nail from the aerosol, which reduces the tackiness of the enamel and prevents smearing if the enamel is touched before being completely dry.

The selection of enamels

A very wide range of coloured enamels is available from the palest of pinks through to the deepest reds. Colour selection is entirely dependant on the client's preference, although the manicurist may need to offer advice regarding colour combination and the suitability of the nail enamel to be used. Crystalline enamels are not recommended for problem nails which are subject to flaking, splitting or ridging. These enamels have a tendency to dry the nail and emphasise any imperfections of the nail plate.

As a general guide, the nail enamel should be harmonious with both the client's make-up and the colour of her clothes. For example, if an orange-toned lipstick is worn, an orange-toned enamel should be chosen. Similarly, a pink lipstick with a blue tone is always complemented by a sugar-pink nail enamel. The colour of the client's skin should also be taken into account. Any shade of enamel looks well on pale skin, while red, bronze and copper tones suit dark skin and bright colours complement sallow skin. Older mature hands tend to look better with subtle, soft dusky shades as opposed to darker vibrant colours.

Faults in enamelling

Incorrect usage of enamels may lead to the subsequent chipping or peeling of the enamel from the nail plate.
Chipping of the enamel may have the following causes:
1. The use of enamel of an incorrect consistency due to over-thinning with nail enamel solvent.

2. Failure to use a base coat.
3. Drying the enamel too quickly, possibly by the use of heat.
4. Failure to 'squeak' the nails before enamelling.
5. The flaking of the nail plates themselves.
   Peeling of the enamel may be due to the following:
1. The use of enamel of incorrect consistency due to thickening by evaporation of the solvent.
2. Failure to use a top coat on a cream enamel.
3. Failure to allow one coat to dry before applying further coats.
4. Failure to 'squeak' the nails before enamelling.

The storage and care of enamels

Nail enamels should be stored in a cool dark place to avoid the possibility of deterioration and fading. The outside of the bottle and its rim should be kept free from enamel not only for the sake of appearance, but also because enamel drying on the rim after the cap has been replaced may make the bottle difficult to open. Alternatively, if the enamel dries on the rim before the cap is replaced, the bottle may no longer be airtight and evaporation of the solvent may occur during storage. If necessary, the rim may be wiped over with a piece of cotton wool moistened with enamel remover. When not in actual use, bottles should always be stoppered to prevent premature evaporation of the solvents which would lead to thickening of the enamel. If by careless use the enamel dries out either wholly or partially, enamel solvent or thinners supplied by the manufacturer should be used to re-dissolve the film-former. This will ensure the correct blend of solvents to restore the drying properties of that particular enamel. The use of nail enamel remover as a thinner, while re-dissolving the enamel, will not restore the correct balance of solvents and drying time may be affected. Nail enamel removers also contain oils such as castor oil or mineral oil which may affect the enamel film and the drying time.

Nail enamel solvent (thinners)

This is used to restore enamels to the correct consistency if they have been allowed to thicken or dry out. Since it should contain the same blend of solvents as originally present in the enamel, it is advisable to use a product made by the same manufacturer. The thinner should be added at least 20 minutes before use to ensure that the enamel is of an even consistency.

Nail enamel remover

Enamel removers are used to re-dissolve the enamel from the nail plate so that it is easily wiped away. They are available as either liquids or creams.

Liquid removers contain mixtures of solvents such as amyl acetate, ethyl acetate and butyl acetate, with castor oil added as an emollient to counteract the drying effect of the solvents. Acetone is now rarely used as a solvent, since it is considered to be too de-greasing to the nail and surrounding skin.

Cream enamel removers are oil-in-water emulsions with castor oil, mineral oil or lanolin in the oil phase, and solvents such as ethyl acetate or butyl acetate in the water phase. Cream removers are less de-greasing than the liquid types.

Paste polish (buffing powders)

Buffing is carried out using a chamois leather pad and a buffing powder containing finely divided talc, kaolin or stannic oxide. The latter is considered the most efficient, but is also the most expensive. The polishes may be prepared in liquid form by suspending the buffing powder in methyl cellulose or gum tragacanth. Alternatively, they may be pressed into a paste polish. Wax polishing sticks are also available and contain carnauba wax and stannic oxide.

Buffing is used for several reasons:
1. To give sheen to the nails if enamel is not to be worn. Buffing is used as an alternative to nail enamel in men's manicure. Certain clients, such as those employed in the food industry and in medical work, may be debarred from using nail enamel due to their occupation. Buffing is also an alternative for clients who are allergic to nail enamels.
2. To even out any ridges on the nail plate by its slightly abrasive action. This gives a smooth base for the application of enamel.
3. To increase the blood flow to the nail, so encouraging growth.

Pumice

Pumice is of volcanic origin and may be in the form of a grey abrasive powder or a rough porous stone. The powder is more abrasive than talc, kaolin or stannic oxide, and may be used in buffing to reduce excessive ridging of the nails. Pumice stone is used to smooth hard skin in the nail area, and to remove tobacco stains from the fingers.

Nail whiteners

These are used under the free edge of the nail to give a clean, white, opaque appearance to the margin of the nail plate. They are not used if coloured enamel is to be extended to the tip of the nail plate, but may be used if clear enamel is to be applied.

The whitener may be in the form of a stiff paste containing a soap base along with a white pigment such as titanium dioxide. Nail white pencils are also available. These contain beeswax, castor oil, cocoa butter, lanolin and titanium dioxide.

Nail bleaches

These may be used for whitening under the free edge, or to remove nicotine stains from the nails and surrounding skin. They are usually formulated as creams or pastes which contain titanium dioxide, talc, mineral oils, petroleum jelly and zinc peroxide.

Nail strengtheners

Nail strengtheners or hardeners are used to counteract fragile or brittle nails. They may contain formaldehyde resin or polyester resin which is applied to the nail before the base coat. Formaldehyde resin is a known sensitiser and may cause allergic reaction in certain people. Alternatively, fine particles of keratin or minute fibres of nylon are incorporated with hard base coat enamels to give support to brittle nails and prevent breakage.

Cuticle massage cream

To restore oil to the skin surrounding the nail and to the nail plate itself, cuticle cream may be applied to the cuticle area as a massage cream during manicure or as a conditioning cream at night. The creams are oil-in-water emulsions containing mineral oil, cocoa butter and lanolin. Oil-soluble vitamins (A, D and E) are sometimes added, though absorption of these is limited since they are applied to only a very small area of the skin.

Cuticle remover (cuticle milk)

Traditionally, cuticle removers contained 2–5 per cent of potassium hydroxide or sodium hydroxide dissolved in water or in a mixture of alcohol and water. These hydroxides are caustic alkalis which soften and destroy keratin; they also remove oils from the skin, so are very drying. Less alkaline products such as triethanolamine or trisodium phosphate are now preferred, though these are slightly less effective than sodium or potassium hydroxide. Glycerol is added as an emollient, and the product is thickened by the addition of gum tragacanth or methyl cellulose.

Questions

1. Explain why the use of nail enamel remover is not recommended for the thinning of nail enamels.
2. What are the qualities of a good nail enamel? How does this affect the choice of materials used in the manufacture of enamels?

3. Explain why:
   (a) nail enamel should be stored in a cool dark place;
   (b) carnauba wax is added to base coat enamels during manufacture;
   (c) crystalline enamels should not be used on brittle or ridged nails.
4. What is the main difference in composition between a cream enamel and a crystalline enamel?
5. In which manicure products would each of the following substances be used?
   (a) triethanolamine
   (b) stannic oxide
   (c) formaldehyde resin

Chapter 19

Manicuring

Manicuring is carried out to enhance and beautify the nails and hands. It involves cleaning and shaping the nails, hand massage, care of the cuticles and the application of nail enamels. The procedure should be carried out in hygienic surroundings and should always be a relaxed and soothing process. Manicurists must create a good impression on their clients by being smart and well groomed. It is essential that manicurists themselves have perfectly manicured hands and nails.

Manicure tools and their use

Tools are required for shaping and polishing the nails, and for carrying out cuticle work.

Emery boards
These are used for filing the nails to shape them, to slightly reduce their length, to bevel the free edges and to remove any barbs. There are various sizes of board, but the professional manicurist normally uses the largest size which is approximately 15 cm in length. For ease of manipulation, the emery board should be quite flexible. One side of the board is coarse and the other side fine. The fine side only is used in ladies' manicure, the coarse side being used for pedicure and in manicure for men.

The emery board should be held at an angle of 45° to the free edge. It is used in one direction only, from the sides of the nail to the centre, and not in a sawing action as the friction produced by this method causes flaking. Nor should nails be filed too deeply into the corners, and a margin of 1–2 mm must be left as a bridge to prevent weakening of the sides of the nail. Weakening of the nail also occurs if filed to a point, and this may lead to splitting and breakage. A new emery board is required for each client.

Nail scissors
These should be extremely sharp and should preferably be made of stainless steel. They are used only for cutting long nails when a much shorter length is required. When reducing the nail length with scissors, allowance should be made for the filing and shaping which follows. The

nails should thus be cut to a length slightly greater than that finally required. Cutting off the excess length is facilitated if the manicurist first flattens the client's nail by applying slight pressure to the nail plate with her thumb. The points of the scissors only should be used.

Orange sticks

As the name implies, these are made of orange wood which is pliable and fine-grained. One end of the stick is sharply pointed, the other being narrow and flat or hoof-shaped. Sterile orange sticks are used to remove preparations such as cuticle massage creams and buffer paste polish from their containers on to the nails. The pointed end, when wrapped in sterile cotton wool, is used for cleaning under the free edge. The hoofed end is used for cuticle work and is always wrapped in sterile cotton wool to afford protection to the cuticles. This is known as a protected orange stick.

Rubber-hoofed orange stick

This orange stick is similar to that mentioned above except that, in this case, the hoofed end is protected by a rubber coating which precludes the need for protection by cotton wool. Its uses are the same as above.

Buffer (see Fig. 19.1)

This may be made of plastic or bone and, apart from the handle, is covered with chamois leather forming a slightly convex pad. On some

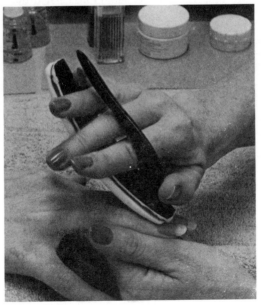

Fig. 19.1 Buffer

buffers the pad of chamois leather is detachable for renewal. The buffer is used with paste polish to give the nails a sheen, stimulate the blood circulation and smooth any surface irregularities. The buffer should be sterilised before use.

Buffing should be carried out in one direction only, from the base of the nail to the free edge. This movement should be smooth but firm and not erratic. Care should be taken to avoid contact of the buffer with the finger joints and skin, and to avoid banging the free edge of the nail.

Cuticle nippers

These are small sharp stainless steel clippers used to nip away excess cuticle. The nails must be dry during this process, and only the points of the nippers used. Extreme care must be taken to avoid nipping the client's skin.

Cuticle knife

A cuticle knife may or may not be required, according to the manicurist's preference. It is used to scrape off any small pieces of cuticle which are adhering to the nail plate after cuticle nipping has taken place. Before use of the knife, the nails should be wetted either with cuticle remover or water. The knife is then held flat on the nail in a horizontal position with the blade pointing away from the flesh (see Fig. 19.2), and is gently used in small circular movements down the nail towards the free edge. The blade must never be angled as otherwise the nail may be damaged by removing layers of the nail plate. The knife should be sharp, and sterilised before use. The process should be carried out with extreme caution.

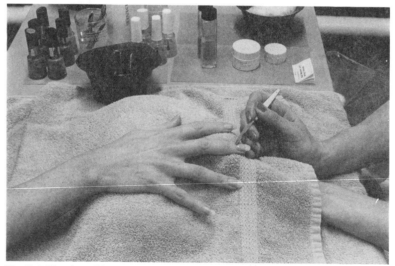

Fig. 19.2 Use of a cuticle knife

Cuticle trimmer

The trimmer has a stainless steel blade with a plastic handle and is used to remove excess cuticle. In practice, it is seldom used as undue pressure is occasionally required on the matrix which may cause ridging of the nails.

Points of hygiene

1. The manicurist's hands should be washed before preparing the equipment, and again both before and after carrying out any manicure treatment.
2. Equipment such as orange sticks, emery boards and cuticle tools should be sterilised before use and kept in an ultra-violet cabinet until required (see Fig. 19.3).

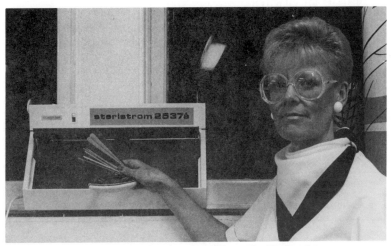

Fig. 19.3 Placing tools in a UV cabinet (courtesy of Coast Air of Sudbury)

3. A sterile orange stick, and not the manicurist's fingers, should be used to remove cosmetic preparations from pots and jars. To avoid cross-infection, a fresh orange stick must be used if additional material is required, and after use on a client the stick should never be re-inserted into any manicure preparation. Soiled sticks should be discarded and never re-used.
4. Soiled cotton wool should be placed in a container and disposed of at the end of the manicure.
5. Extreme care should be taken not to damage or puncture the skin and nails when using sharp or pointed tools. If during manicure the client is inadvertently cut, antiseptic should be applied immediately. Any blood on the tool should be washed off, the tool wiped with surgical spirit, and re-sterilised immediately. The manicurist should, as far as

Record card for manicure

Name of client.....................................

Address...

....

....

Tel. no ....

Name of doctor.....................................

Address...

....

....

Contra-indications ....

....

Date	Treatment	Remarks	Manicurist

Fig. 19.4 Record card (manicure)

possible, prevent the client's blood from coming into contact with her own hands.

Contra-indications to manicure

1. Infection of the skin surrounding the nails.
2. Nail diseases and disorders.
3. Bruised nails.
4. Cuts and abrasions of the surrounding skin.
5. Recent scar tissue in the surrounding skin.
6. Allergy to products.

Use of record card

It is an essential part of the work of a manicurist to keep a record card for each client concerning the manicure treatment given. A typical card is shown in Fig. 19.4.

Manicure techniques

1. Finger rotation
The manicure procedure will differ slightly according to whether the manicurist is right-handed or left-handed. The finger rotation, or sequence in which the fingers are treated during the manicure procedure, must be carried out methodically according to the dexterity of the manicurist, as shown in Fig. 19.5. This will prevent the manicurist from becoming confused as to which fingers have been treated during the manicure, and reduce the possibility of smudging or spoiling the nail enamel application. The same finger rotation is employed throughout all the stages of the manicure including removal of enamel, shaping the nails, buffing, cuticle work, hand massage and nail enamelling.

2. Cuticle work
The cuticle is a modification of the stratum corneum of the nail fold which grows on to the nail plate. Its function is to protect the nail matrix from infection by sealing the nail fold. As the cuticle adheres firmly to the nail plate it may become over-stretched and crack as the nail grows forwards. During manicure, this outer edge of the cuticle is released from the nail plate and excess removed, but the seal itself must not be broken. The removal of excess cuticle is carried out primarily for aesthetic reasons because it gives a cleaner appearance and better shape to the nail plate. However, extreme care should always be taken to avoid puncturing the client's skin or damaging the nail plate. The use of chemical cuticle removers is thus preferable to the use of cutting tools.

Sequence of finger rotation for manicure

Sequence for **left-handed** manicurists	Sequence for **right-handed** manicurists
1. Start with the client's **left** hand	1. Start with the client's **left** hand
Order of working 1. Thumb 2. Little finger 3. Ring finger 4. Middle finger 5. Index finger	*Order of working* 1. Thumb 2. Index finger 3. Middle finger 4. Ring finger 5. Little finger
2. Progress to the client's **right** hand	2. Progress to the client's **right** hand.
Order of working 1. Thumb 2. Index finger 3. Middle finger 4. Ring finger 5. Little finger	*Order of working* 1. Thumb 2. Little finger 3. Ring finger 4. Middle finger 5. Index finger
This sequence should be followed throughout the manicure	This sequence should be followed throughout the manicure

Fig. 19.5 Finger rotation for manicure

Corrective work on the cuticles should never be carried out unless they have been softened by the application of cuticle massage cream, and the fingers then soaked in warm water to aid penetration of the cream into the cuticles. After drying the hands, cuticle remover is applied. This contains a caustic alkali which will further soften the cuticles. They can then be moulded back with the hoofed end of a protected orange stick without using excessive pressure. The caustic cuticle remover must be thoroughly rinsed off as soon as moulding back is completed, to avoid damage to the cuticles.

The loosened cuticles can then be assessed. Cutting tools must only be employed if there is excess cuticle to be trimmed. If necessary, trimming may be carried out using cuticle nippers and for this procedure the nails must be dry. Any remaining cuticle adhering to the nail may then be removed using a cuticle knife, and in this case the nails must be wet. A cuticle trimmer may also be used but this implement requires a certain amount of pressure to be exerted on the matrix, and may result in ridged nails. The manicurist may develop a preference for one or more of the cutting tools and may not necessarily use them all.

3. Nail enamel application
It is usual to apply four coats of enamel to the nails. If cream enamel is to be used, the four coats consist of a base coat, two coats of cream enamel and a top coat. The use of two coats of cream enamel gives a better depth of colour and a better finish, as the first coat tends to look rather transparent and may be streaky. The use of a top coat adds sheen. For crystalline enamels, a base coat and three coats of crystalline enamel are required, with no top coat since this type of enamel is already glossy.

Nail enamelling is usually carried out so that the whole nail is covered by the enamel. However, certain clients may require the application to be carried out leaving the entire half moon area free from enamel. This is often used to make the nails look longer, or may be merely a fashion trend. The application is then much more difficult since an even and clean line round the half moon is required.

Preparation of equipment

The following equipment and materials are required when setting up a manicure table. Bottles and jars should be free from spills and drips and tidily arranged, before the arrival of the client.

Emery boards ⎫
Orange sticks ⎪
Cuticle nippers ⎬ These items should be kept in a UV cabinet until required
Cuticle knife ⎪
Buffer ⎭

A waste bowl
A water bowl
Cotton wool and container
Liquid soap
Cuticle massage cream
Cuticle remover
Base coat
Top coat
Paste polish
Selection of crystalline enamels
Selection of cream enamels
Nail enamel solvent
Nail enamel remover
Hand cream
Nail repair tissues
Nail cement

The manicurist needs access to a UV cabinet and an adequate supply of both hot and cold water. A table or trolley from which to work and to hold the manicure preparations should also be available, along with two chairs suitable for the manicurist and the client. To avoid fatigue and discomfort, it is essential that the manicurist is able to work at a comfortable height without having to stoop or bend too much. The table should be laid out with three towels. One is placed lengthwise across the table between the manicurist and client. A second is folded to form a pad on which to rest the client's hand while work is in progress (a cushion may be used instead). The third is folded in half widthways and placed across the table over the pad, with the open ends facing the manicurist whose hands are easily slipped in between the folds in order to dry the client's hand or to give support during cuticle work. A fourth towel is placed across the manicurist's knees for use during the manicure.

The correct layout and preparation of the manicure table is crucial in order to carry out an efficient and methodical manicure. If the manicurist is right-handed, then all the required materials are placed on a table to the right for easy access and to avoid having to reach over during the manicure (see Fig. 19.6). If left-handed, the table and materials would be to the left.

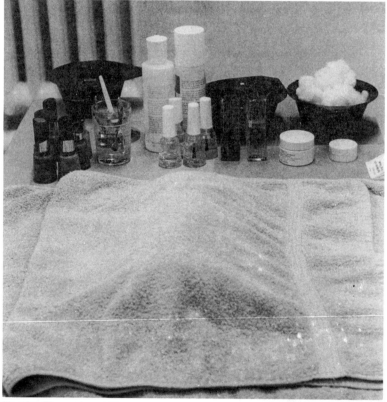

Fig. 19.6 The manicure table

Preparation of the client

1. Ensure that the client is seated comfortably, facing directly opposite to the manicurist.
2. Ask the client to remove any jewellery worn on the hands, and help her to turn back her sleeves away from the wrists.
3. Inspect the client's hands carefully for any conditions which would be contra-indicative to manicure. If any nail or skin infection is present, the manicure must not proceed and the client should be advised to seek medical attention.
4. Note the shape and length of the nails in order to assess the amount of shaping required and discuss this with the client. Ask the client also to select the colour of enamel required.

Manicure procedure

Manicure may be carried out on both male and female clients. The procedure is the same in each case, though male clients would not normally require nail enamel. Before commencing the manicure, a final check of the equipment and materials should be made to avoid leaving the client once treatment has begun. In particular, the nail enamel should be checked for correct consistency; if necessary, it should be thinned with a little enamel solvent.

1. Cleansing the client's hands
Using an antiseptic solution such as cetrimide or surgical spirit on a cotton wool ball (see Fig. 19.7), cleanse the client's hands thoroughly. (Cotton wool balls should always be held firmly between the index finger and the second finger about half way up the fingers on the working hand.)

2. Removal of old enamel
Dry the client's hands if necessary. Hold a cotton wool ball in the manner previously described (this prevents the unwanted removal of the manicurist's own enamel), and pour a little enamel remover directly from the bottle on to the cotton wool. Place the ball firmly on the nail being worked on, while supporting the underside of the finger with your thumb (see Fig. 19.8). Gently rock the cotton wool from side to side on the nail to allow the remover to dissolve the old enamel. Slide the cotton wool ball down the nail, removing the enamel as you do so. Treat all the fingers in the same way, using clean cotton wool as necessary and following the finger rotation procedure according to your dexterity. For the removal of dark enamels a clean piece of cotton wool may be required for each nail, to prevent the staining of the skin. Finally, remove any stubborn areas of enamel around the cuticles and nail walls, using a

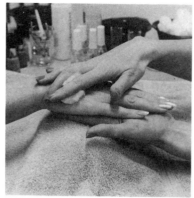

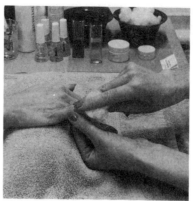

Fig. 19.7 Cleansing the client's hands   **Fig. 19.8** Removing the enamel

sterile orange stick protected by cotton wool impregnated with remover, by gently rolling the orange stick along the cuticle and the nail walls.

3. Re-examination of the hands

At this stage, since all the enamel has been removed, it is possible to scrutinise the nails more closely in order to detect any imperfections previously hidden by the enamel. The necessary work may therefore be re-assessed.

4. Shaping the nails (left-hand nails only)

Take the client's left hand and, using the finger rotation as shown in Fig. 19.5, commence to shape the nails by use of the fine side of a flexible emery board (see Fig. 19.9). Start at one side of the nail and work to the centre. Then change to the opposite side and again work to the centre of the nail using firm single strokes at all times. (Never use a sawing action

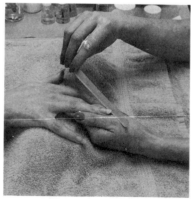

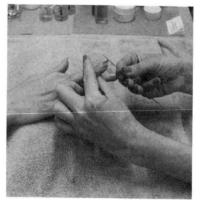

Fig. 19.9 Shaping the nails   **Fig. 19.10** Bevelling

as the to and fro movement tends to loosen the nail from the nail bed.) Some nails may require more shaping than others depending on the frequency of previous manicures, but the intended shape should be oval. Always ensure an even shape, making sure that the sides of the nail are symmetrical. Finish the shaping by drawing the fine side of the emery board down over the end of the free edge to remove any unevenness. This technique is known as bevelling (see Fig. 19.10). Follow the same procedure on each of the other fingers of the left hand.

5. Buffing (left-hand nails only)
Using the pointed end of a sterile orange stick, remove a small amount of paste polish from the container, sufficient to dot on each nail of the left hand. Using the index finger, gently smooth the paste over the nails ensuring that it only covers the nail plates. Using a sterilised buffer, buff each nail plate by placing the buffer at the base of the nail and drawing it down to the free edge using smooth even strokes. Six to eight strokes per nail should be sufficient to produce a good sheen. Always buff in the same direction and never bang the buffer down on to the nail plate (see Fig. 19.11).

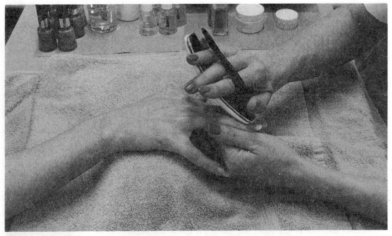

Fig. 19.11 Buffing

6. Cuticle massage (left-hand nails only)
Using a sterile orange stick, remove sufficient cuticle massage cream from the pot to use on all five nails. Place the cream on the cuticle of each nail by rolling the orange stick against them, thus depositing enough cream for the massage (see Fig. 19.12(a)). Using both hands, take the client's hand and massage the cream into the cuticles with a rotary movement. Then place the client's hand in a bowl of warm water containing a small quantity of liquid soap (see Fig. 19.12(b)).

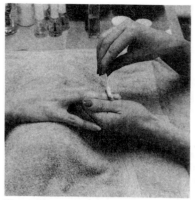

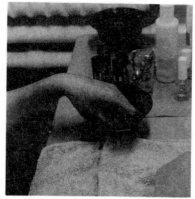

Fig. 19.12(a) Application of cuticle massage cream

Fig. 19.12(b) Client's fingers in bowl of water

7. *Treatment of the right-hand nails*

Now with the client's right hand, repeat the procedure from point no 4. to point no. 6 to shape and buff the nails and massage the cuticles.

8. *Moulding back the cuticles* (see Fig. 19.13)

Remove the left hand from the bowl of water and dry it gently. Next apply cuticle remover to the left hand using the brush provided with the remover. Four strokes of the brush are required: one stroke is made down each side of the nail, one across the base and the fourth under the free edge. Carry out this procedure on all five nails. Using a sterile protected orange stick impregnated with cuticle remover, clean under the free edge of each nail (see Fig. 19.14). Change the cotton wool and with the hoofed end of the orange stick gently mould back the cuticles and the sides of the nail. It is important to use the hoofed end only and to avoid undue pressure, as otherwise damage may occur.

Remove the client's right hand from the water and dry it gently. Place

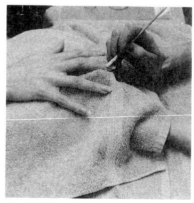

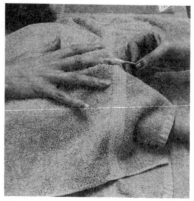

Fig. 19.13 Moulding back the cuticle

Fig. 19.14 Cleansing under the free edge

the client's left hand in the water and remove all traces of cuticle remover by sponging down each nail with a ball of cotton wool, and paying particular attention to the underside of the free edge. Remove the hand from the water and dry it.

Apply cuticle remover to the right hand, repeating the procedure as above.

9. Cutting back excess cuticle (see Fig. 19.15)
If excess cuticle is present, it may be cut back using cuticle nippers. Only the points of the nippers must be used and the nails must be dry. Any remaining cuticle left adhering to the nail plate may be removed using a cuticle knife on a wet nail. Extreme care is needed when using these cutting tools. (Refer also to details of cuticle work given earlier in this chapter under 'Manicure techniques'.)

10. Hand massage
Apply hand cream and then massage the left hand first. Details of the procedure are given in Chapter 20. Then repeat for the right-hand massage.

11. 'Squeaking' the nails (see Fig. 19.16)
Hold a clean ball of cotton wool impregnated with nail enamel remover firmly between the index finger and the second finger. Using a firm stroking action, 'squeak' the nails by drawing the cotton wool ball once down each nail. This removes any grease and prepares the nail for the enamel. If there is a long free edge, remove any grease from behind the nail using a protected orange stick and enamel remover. Work first on the left hand then on the right.

12. Nail repairs
At this stage any nail repairs may be carried out if required. These are described in detail in Chapter 22.

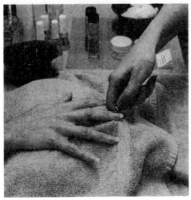
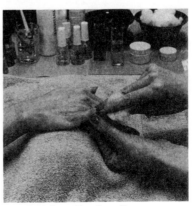

Fig. 19.15 Use of cuticle nippers   **Fig. 19.16** Squeaking the nails

13. *Application of base coat*

The client's rings may be replaced at this stage before enamelling takes place. With a brush and again using the correct finger rotation, apply the base coat to the nails of the left hand, ensuring that it is kept off the skin. For evenness of application, use three brush strokes down the length of the nail from the cuticle to the free edge, starting with a centre stroke followed by one stroke on either side. Repeat the application on the nails of the right hand.

14. *Application of nail enamel* (see Fig. 19.17)

When the base coat is dry, apply the nail enamel in the same manner, first to the left-hand nails and then to the right-hand nails. Avoid flooding the enamel in the cuticle area, which may be caused by excess enamel on the applicator brush. Two coats of cream enamel are required, or three coats if crystalline enamel is being used. Each coat should be allowed to dry before applying another, as otherwise peeling of the enamel may occur later.

While enamelling is in progress, an unprotected sterile orange stick should be kept in a bottle of enamel remover ready for use in case any staining of the skin occurs. Any spots of enamel on the skin can then be gently wiped away with the orange stick before they dry.

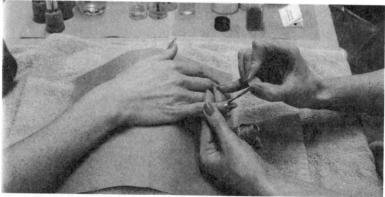

Fig. 19.17 Application of enamel

15. *Application of top coat*

Finally, if cream enamels have been used, a top coat is applied to add sheen. This is not required over crystalline enamels.

16. *Drying the enamel*

In order to speed the drying of the nails, nail enamel dryer may be sprayed across them from an aerosol can (see Fig. 19.18).

Ask the client to rest the hand and relax for a few minutes to allow the

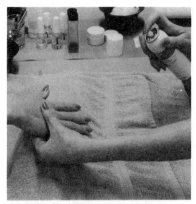

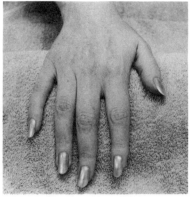

Fig. 19.18 Drying the enamel using an aerosol spray

Fig. 19.19 The completed manicure

nails to dry completely and to prevent smudging the enamel. The manicure procedure is then completed (see Fig. 19.19).

The care of the hands and nails

On completion of the manicure, advice should, if necessary, be given to the client on the care of the hands so that they may be kept in good condition. This mainly involves the maintenance of an oily layer on the skin which helps to keep it supple by retaining moisture in the stratum corneum, so enabling the skin to stretch and wrinkle without cracking. If the oily layer is absent, soaking the hands in water may result in it entering the horny layer, causing swelling of the tissues. Groups of cells may thus be dislodged causing roughness of the skin surface and possible chapping when the skin is dried. Bacteria may infect the small cracks in the skin, resulting in inflammation.

To keep the hands in good condition

1. Excessive use of detergents, which degrease the skin and nails, should be avoided.
2. Rubber or plastic gloves should be worn whenever the hands are to be immersed in water for some time. If the use of gloves is impossible due to allergy to rubber or is inconvenient, barrier creams should be used as an alternative. Barrier creams are water-in-oil emulsions containing mineral oils with a small proportion of silicone oils which are water-repellant.
3. Hand creams should be applied on drying the hands after the use of water and detergents. These may be light non-greasy creams of the moisturising type.

4. Hand creams should also be used at night. Hand massage creams with a higher oil content may be beneficial if the skin is rough.
5. Detergents left on the skin may cause dermatitis. Care should be taken to rinse the skin well after their use, particularly between the fingers and under rings.
6. Protective gloves should be worn for all dirty, dry work such as gardening.
7. Gloves should be worn for warmth in cold weather to maintain adequate blood circulation to the hands and nails, so preventing chapping and the development of chilblains.

Questions

1. Describe the correct method for buffing the nails. Explain why (a) buffing is sometimes preferred by a client as an alternative to the use of nail enamel and (b) buffing is beneficial for ridged nails.
2. What is the cause of nail enamel streaking on application?
3. Explain the use of the coarse side and the fine side of an emery board. In what ways may incorrect filing damage the nails.
4. Explain why a client's hands should be closely inspected before carrying out a manicure.
5. What precautions should be taken in the use of cuticle-cutting tools during a manicure? Why is cuticle nipping not always advisable when carrying out a manicure?

Chapter 20

Massage of the hand and wrist

The purpose of hand and wrist massage is to improve the circulation of the blood to the skin and nails, to soften the skin by removal of loose keratin scales from the surface, and to increase the mobility of the joints. A knowledge of the anatomy of the area will assist the manicurist to give maximum benefit to the client during the massage treatment.

The anatomy of the forearm, wrist and hand

The complicated movements of which the hand is capable depend on the bone structure of the wrist and hand, and on the muscles which control the movement of those bones. There are few muscles in the hand itself, most of those responsible for hand movements being situated in the forearm and connected to the hand by long tendons. Thus the hand itself is slim, and this facilitates both the grasping of objects and the fine movements of which it is capable. The many small bones (eight in the wrist and nineteen in the hand), and hence the large number of joints between the bones, enables a wide range of hand movements to be performed.

The bone structure of the forearm, wrist and hand

The bones of this area are shown and named in Fig. 20.1.

The forearm consists of two long bones, the radius and ulna. At their upper end they articulate with the humerus bone in the upper arm to form a hinge joint at the elbow, enabling the arm to be bent and straightened. The radius, the smaller of the forearm bones, is on the thumb side of the arm and at its lower end articulates with the bones of the wrist. The ulna, on the little finger side of the forearm, articulates only with the radius and is separated from the wrist by a pad of cartilage.

The bones of the wrist, the carpus, consist of a group of eight small irregularly-shaped carpal bones arranged in two rows of four. The bones are held together by ligaments. Gliding joints between the bones allow them to slide over each other to permit slight movement. The upper row forms a double hinge joint with the radius allowing a wide range of movement at this joint. The lower row, nearest the hand, forms gliding joints with the metacarpal bones of the hand so that movement here is

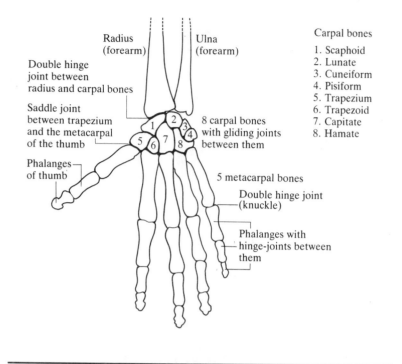

Fig. 20.1 Bones of the forearm, wrist and hand

limited, except in the case of the metacarpal for the thumb which is attached to the trapezium bone of the wrist in a saddle joint and allows a wide range of movement (like the rider on a horse).

The hand contains five metacarpal bones (together called the metacarpus) which run along the palm of the hand and articulate with the bones of the digits (the fingers and thumb) in double hinge joints. The rounded heads of the metacarpals form the knuckles. The four metacarpals attached to the bones of the fingers are almost parallel to each other, but the metacarpal attached to the thumb is shorter and is set at an angle. The thumb itself consists of two bones while each finger has three bones. The bones (phalanges) for each digit are connected by hinge joints which allow movement in one direction only, like the hinge of a door.

The muscles of the forearm and hand

The muscles of the forearm and hand are shown in Fig. 20.2. The long tendons which move the fingers run from the arm muscles to the bones of the finger tips. By placing the hand palm downwards on a flat surface and raising the fingers, the tendons may be felt along the back of the hand. These are known as extensor tendons and are used to straighten the fingers by contraction of the extensor muscles in the arm. Running along the palm of the hand are the flexor tendons which are used to close the fingers, as in gripping an object in the palm of the hand. The tendons of the arm muscles are bound down by the circular ligament just above the wrist joint.

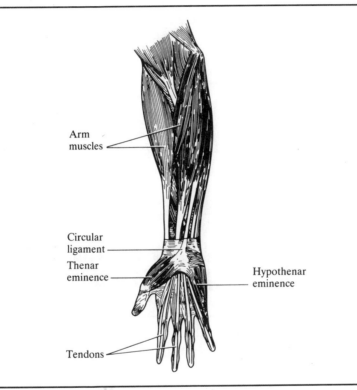

Fig. 20.2 Muscles of the forearm and hand

The muscles of the hand itself consist of a short flexor muscle for the thumb, and small muscles to enable the fingers to move from side to side. These are most prominent on the palm of the hand at the base of the thumb (the thenar eminence) and at the base of the little finger (the hypothenar eminence).

The blood supply to the arm and hand

The arterial blood supply to the hand, which carries nutrients and oxygen to the tissues, is shown in Fig. 20.3. The radial and ulna arteries of the forearm each divide at the wrist. The two branches curve to meet each other forming the palmar arches, one deep in the hand and the other close to the surface of the palm. Smaller digital arteries branch from the arches to the fingers, adjacent surfaces of the fingers being supplied from the same small artery.

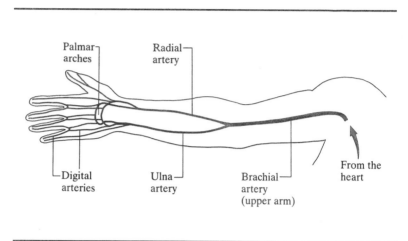

Fig. 20.3 Arteries of the forearm and hand

The blood is drained from the hand in a network of veins, which join to form the three main veins of the forearm (the cephalic, median and basilic veins) and carry blood back towards the heart (see Fig. 20.4).

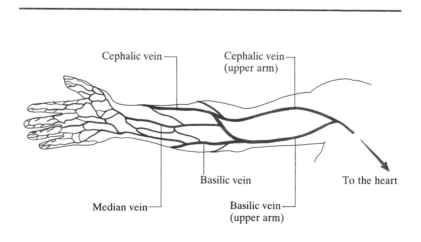

Fig. 20.4 Veins of the forearm and hand

Hand massage

All massage techniques should be pleasant, soothing and relaxing. Numerous methods of carrying out massage are possible, and many manicurists adapt techniques to create their own sequence of movements.

Massage movements

During hand and wrist massage, a combination of effleurage, petrissage, tapotement and light friction movements are used, the massage being carried out from the finger tips to the wrist. The movements should be smooth, and a fluent but firm manipulation is essential.

Effleurage is a gentle stroking movement. It is often used at the beginning or end of the treatment, and also between more vigorous movements since it has a soothing and relaxing effect.

Petrissage involves circular movements using the thumbs or finger tips to apply pressure in a kneading action.

Tapotement is a percussion movement involving a light tapping action by the fingers.

Friction movements are small circular or 'to and fro' movements in which the skin is moved under the first two fingers or the thumb.

Hand creams and lotions

Hand massage during manicure is always carried out using a hand cream or lotion to act as a lubricant between the client's skin and the manicurist's hands, so facilitating the flow of massage movements without drag on the skin. The creams are usually oil-in-water emulsions similar to moisturising creams, so should rub in easily leaving the skin soft and non-greasy. They may contain stearic acid, lanolin, mineral oil, cetyl alcohol, glycerol and water. Lotions may contain the same ingredients as hand creams but have a greater proportion of water. Creams usually contain about 30 per cent of oily substances and 70 per cent of water, while lotions have about 15 per cent of oily substances and 85 per cent of water. The use of an excessive amount of cream should be avoided as otherwise the massage movements would be difficult to carry out.

Massage procedure

Massage takes place after any cuticle work has been carried out. The client should be seated comfortably and the manicurist's hands should be spotlessly clean.

1. Pour sufficient hand cream into the palm of your hand to carry out the massage of the client's left hand, then spread the cream evenly over the palms of both your hands.
2. Support the client's hand with the palm of your right hand, and place

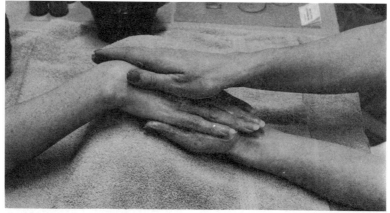

Fig. 20.5 Effleurage to smooth in the cream

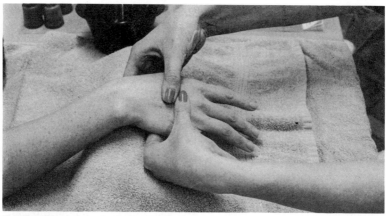

Fig. 20.6 Petrissage on the back of the hand

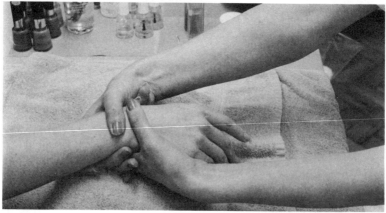

Fig. 20.7 Friction movements round the wrist

the palm of the left hand over the top of the client's hand. Then proceed to smooth in the cream by using an effleurage (stroking) action (see Fig. 20.5).

3. Place the thumbs on the back of the client's hand, supporting the palm with the fingers. Carry out petrissage movements using a rotary action, following a figure of eight movement over the entire back of the hand (see Fig. 20.6).
4. Using both hands, span the client's wrist and carry out friction movements, rotating around the wrist, (see Fig. 20.7).
5. Release the wrist and gently slide down each side of the hand, one hand taking hold of the little finger and the other grasping the thumb.
6. Using the thumbs of each hand, carry out a petrissage movement, progressing up the client's little finger and thumb at the same time, using the remaining fingers to give support. When the knuckles are reached, slide back down to the finger tips and repeat the manoeuvre back up to the knuckles and down again 4 or 5 times (see Fig. 20.8).
7. Take hold of the client's ring finger and index finger in exactly the same way, and carry out the same massage movements up to the knuckle. Slide down and repeat this 4 or 5 times.
8. Carry out the same movements on the middle finger and the thumb.
9. Place one thumb at the knuckle of the little finger and the other at the knuckle of the thumb, supporting the palm with the fingers. Using the thumbs, carry out petrissage movements along the line of the metacarpals, again repeating the movements 4 or 5 times (see Fig. 20.9). Using the same sequence as above, massage along the line of the metacarpals above the ring finger and index finger, and then finally along the metacarpals above the middle finger and thumb.
10. Place the thumbs at the centre of the wrist, supporting the underside of the wrist with the fingers. Carry out petrissage movements using a rotary action across the top of the wrist (see Fig. 20.10).
11. Slide down to the finger tips and carry out rotation of the fingers (see Fig. 20.11) using the finger sequence outlined in Fig. 19.5.
12. Place the thumb of one hand under the client's palm and lay the fingers across the knuckles. Using your other hand, take hold of the client's thumb and circle it three times in a clockwise direction, and then three times in an anti-clockwise direction. Following the same procedure, rotate the fingers in turn using the correct finger sequence according to your dexterity. (While this massage is being executed, the movement of the client's joints should be felt by the manicurist's fingers lying across the knuckles.)
13. After ensuring that the client's elbow is resting firmly on the manicure table, interlock your fingers with those of the client and support the wrist with your other hand. Next rotate the wrist three times in a clockwise direction and three times in an anti-clockwise direction (see Fig. 20.12).
14. Finally, while the fingers are still interlocked, lower the client's hand

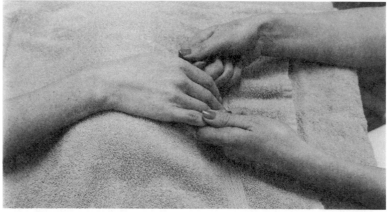

Fig. 20.8 Petrissage along the phalanges

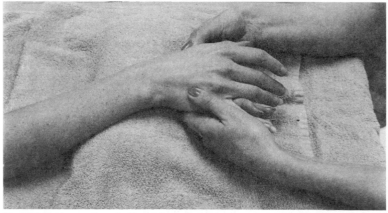

Fig. 20.9 Petrissage along the line of the metacarpals

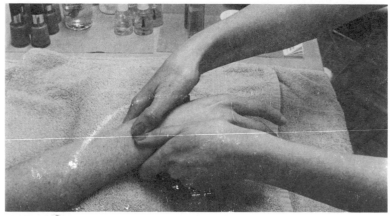

Fig. 20.10 Petrissage across the carpus

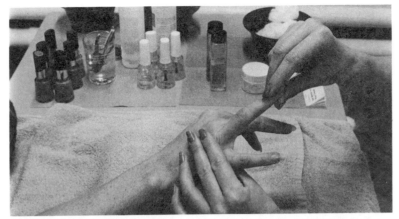

Fig. 20.11 Rotation of the fingers

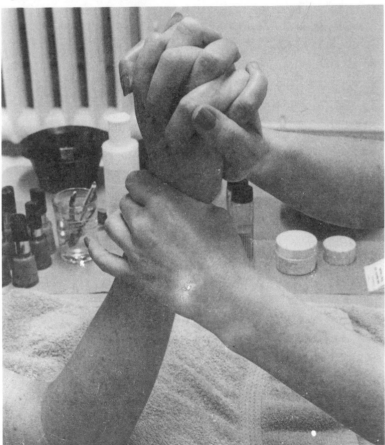

Fig. 20.12 Rotation of the wrist

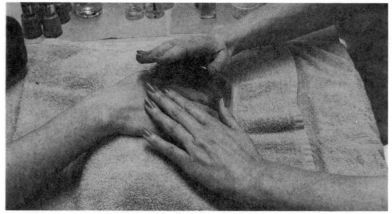

Fig. 20.13 Tapotement on the back of the hand

gently to the pad on the manicure table and withdraw your fingers by sliding them away. Complete the massage by gentle tapotement across the back of the hand and fingers (see Fig. 20.13). Turn the client's hand over and carry out the same gentle tapotement movements across the palm and fingers.
15. Repeat the entire procedure on the client's right hand.

Questions

1. What is the purpose of hand massage in manicure? At what stage of the manicure would hand massage be carried out?
2. State two differences between effleurage and petrissage massage movements as carried out during hand massage.
3. What is the function of hand cream (a) applied during hand massage and (b) applied at night?
4. Name the type of joint (a) between the phalanges and (b) between the carpal bones.
5. Name the two main arteries bringing blood to the wrist and hand. Explain how the two arteries divide to supply blood to the fingers and the nail beds.

Chapter 21

Remedial treatments

When the nails and skin of the hands are in poor condition, remedial treatments may be beneficial. These are carried out as part of the manicure procedure and used at the discretion of the manicurist.

The oil manicure

Oil manicures are particularly beneficial for brittle or ridged nails and dry cuticles. In extreme cases, treatment may be necessary once a month until there is a noticeable change in the condition of the hands and nails. A vegetable oil such as olive oil is used for this treatment as it is capable of penetration and will therefore improve the nails and leave the skin of the hands soft and pliable.

Procedure

1. Warm the vegetable oil in a double saucepan, testing the oil on the back of your own hand to ensure that it is not too hot for client comfort.
2. Follow the usual manicure procedure to complete the shaping and buffing of the nails of the left hand. Do not apply cuticle massage cream but at this stage, having checked the temperature of the oil, place the client's hand in the warm oil.
3. Leave the left hand in the oil while repeating the same stages of manicure on the right hand. Then remove the left hand from the oil and immerse the right hand.
4. Massage the left hand, following the normal massage procedure with correct finger rotation.
5. Using a protected orange stick, mould back the cuticles. (Cuticle remover and massage cream are not required here.)
6. Remove the oil from the hand using a warm steam towel prepared by immersing a clean towel in very hot water and wringing out the excess. The two ends of the towel should be kept dry to allow it to be twisted to expel excess water, without scalding the manicurist's hands.
7. Carry out the same procedure on the client's right hand.

8. When all the oil has been removed, apply a skin freshener to both hands using a pad of cotton wool dampened with freshener.
9. Using nail enamel remover and a ball of cotton wool, wipe over each nail to ensure that all traces of oil are removed before applying the base coat.
10. Complete the manicure following the procedure for the normal manicure, i.e. base coat, enamel, and top coat if rquired.

Paraffin wax treatment

This is a treatment involving the use of warm paraffin wax. It is particularly useful if the skin of the hands is dry, and may be beneficial to the joints of the fingers if stiffness is present. Much of the benefit of the treatment is derived from the build-up of heat within the skin, which in turn brings about relaxation of the hand and fingers.

Procedure

1. Immerse the client's hand for a short time in melted paraffin wax heated to about 48 °C. Alternatively, the wax may be applied with a brush.
2. Allow the wax to solidify on the hand and then re-immerse or re-brush in order to obtain a second coating.
3. When completely solidified but before the hand cools, wrap the coated hand in aluminium foil or polythene, and finally wrap in a warm towel to retain the heat. Leave for 15 minutes.
4. Remove the wrapping materials and peel off the wax. This should come away easily and no further cleaning should be required.

The salt rub

The salt is prepared by mixing it to a paste with a little water. It is applied by means of a spatula and massaged into the skin of the hands. A 5 minute massage is quite adequate and will cause hyperaemia. Thus the salt rub is beneficial for hands with poor circulation. Due to the rough texture of the paste, it would also help to break down calluses. A salt rub should not be used on dry skin since it may aggravate the condition.

The bran bath

This is used on dingy, grimy-looking hands. Massage is carried out before application of the bran. The bran should be mixed to a creamy paste with warm water, or with warm olive oil if the hands are particularly dry. A small amount of lemon juice may be added if the hands are excessively dirty. The bran is applied with a spatula, gently rubbed into the skin and left for ten minutes. It is then removed using warm water and cotton wool.

As an alternative to bran, a paste may be made of magnesium carbonate and water and used in the same way. Fuller's earth mixed with rose water may also be used.

Calamine treatment

It is essential that none of the above treatments are carried out on hands where the skin is broken by cuts or abrasions, since irritation may occur. If minor cuts or irritations are present, a paste may be made with calamine and rose water, and applied before carrying out hand massage. It should be left for ten minutes before being removed with warm water and cotton wool. The treatment is also beneficial for the soothing of rashes.

Questions

1. State the type of oil used when carrying out an oil manicure and give reasons for its use.
2. Which remedial treatment is particularly beneficial for stiffness of the joints and dry skin?
3. Which treatment is recommended for dingy, grimy-looking hands? What ingredient may be added to improve the appearance of excessively dirty hands?
4. What precautions should be taken when carrying out remedial treatments on hands where the skin is broken?
5. At what point in the manicure procedure would an oil manicure be given? Which manicure preparations does the oil replace?

Chapter 22

Nail repairs

Nails may break, split or flake for various reasons. They may be congenitally weak, but the damage is more often caused by misuse such as the over-use of harsh detergents or incorrect filing during manicure. Accidental damage may also occur if long nails are knocked or trapped. Self-inflicted breaks may be caused by the nervous habit of picking at nail enamel or at the nails themselves. Ill-health, poor circulation of blood to the fingers, and lack of vitamins A and B_2 are also contributory causes of weak nails. Fortunately, damaged nails can be repaired and, if done correctly, the repair may be practically invisible. Nails are usually repaired by the tissue method.

Materials used

The repair is carried out using a liquid nail cement and special tissue or mending paper as supplied by a manufacturer. Nail cement or mending solution may consist of methyl methacrylate (a vinyl resin) or may be a base coat enamel thickened by resin. The tissue is shaped to fit the repair, and is saturated with cement before application to the damaged area. Nail enamel solvent is used in smoothing the patch.

Types of repair

Repairs are always carried out after 'squeaking' the nails and before the application of enamels. There are four different types of repair.
(a) The capping of a fragile nail tip.
(b) A split on the free edge of the nail.
(c) A split below the flesh line.
(d) The re-attachment of a broken nail.

Method of capping a fragile tip (see Fig. 22.1)

1. Ensure that the nail surface is clean and free from grease by cleansing it with nail enamel remover.

2. Take a repair tissue and tear off a round piece sufficient to cover the repair and to extend slightly beyond the free edge. (Tearing the tissue enables the repair to be more easily disguised, since no straight edge is left.)
3. Using the brush applicator supplied, apply the liquid cement to the tissue until it is saturated. Next, using an orange stick, place it with the wet side down on to the nail tip, so that the tissue extends slightly beyond the free edge.
4. Turn the client's hand over with the palm uppermost and apply more cement to the exposed edge of the tissue. Using an orange stick dipped in nail enamel solvent, gently turn down the tissue inwards and over the edge of the nail. Press firmly to ensure adhesion of the tissue to the nail.
5. Turn the client's hand over again and with your thumb moistened with nail enamel solvent, gently smooth the patch. Leave for 2–3 minutes to dry thoroughly before applying the base coat and enamel to complete the manicure.

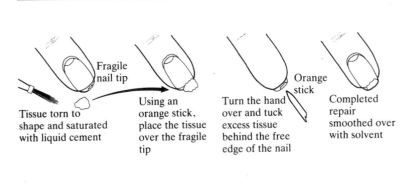

Tissue torn to shape and saturated with liquid cement

Using an orange stick, place the tissue over the fragile tip

Turn the hand over and tuck excess tissue behind the free edge of the nail

Completed repair smoothed over with solvent

Fig. 22.1 Capping a fragile nail tip

To repair a split on the free edge (see Fig. 22.2)

1. Cleanse the nail as before.
2. Tear a small piece of double tissue into a circular shape and saturate it with liquid cement.
3. Using an orange stick, place the tissue over the broken or split area so that it overlaps the edge of the nail.
4. Again using an orange stick, tuck the tissue behind the free edge. Then moisten the thumb with solvent and smooth lightly over the patch.
5. Allow to dry thoroughly before applying the base coat and enamel.

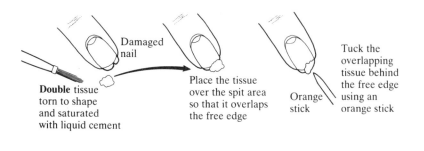

Fig. 22.2 To repair a split on the free edge

To repair a split below the flesh line (see Fig. 22.3)

1. Cleanse the nail with nail enamel remover as before.
2. Take a wisp of cotton wool, saturate it with liquid cement and then lay it flat over the split, allowing it to extend slightly beyond the break.
3. Trim the cotton wool and, using an orange stick, tuck it behind the broken nail.
4. Saturate a strip of tissue with cement and place it diagonally over the cotton wool. Trim the excess tissue leaving sufficient to tuck behind the nail.
5. Using the applicator brush, stipple over the patch with liquid cement.
6. Moisten the thumb with solvent and smooth over the patch in order to make the repair as smooth as possible.
7. Allow to dry thoroughly before applying the base coat and enamel.

Nail with split below the flesh line

Cotton wool saturated with liquid cement placed over the split. Excess trimmed and tucked behind broken nail

Saturated tissue placed over cotton wool. Tissue trimmed and excess tucked behind the nail using an orange stick

Fig. 22.3 To repair a split below the flesh line

To re-attach a broken nail (see Fig. 22.4)

1. Cleanse the nail as before.
2. Take a wisp of cotton wool and saturate it with liquid cement. Place the cotton wool down the centre of the nail leaving a little projecting over the broken free edge.
3. Smooth down the cotton wool with an orange stick soaked in solvent.
4. Apply cement to the edge of the broken off nail tip and place it in position over the cotton wool. Hold the nail firmly in position until the cement sets.
5. Carefully turn the client's hand palm upwards, and trim the cotton wool halfway down the underside of the nail. Gently smooth the cotton wool on the back of the free edge.
6. Turn the client's hand over again and bring the cotton wool up from the cuticle as near to the join as possible, smoothing it away to avoid a hard line.
7. Tear off a small piece of tissue, saturate it with cement and place it horizontally across the repair. Gently smooth over the tissue using solvent on the thumb. Trim both sides of the tissue leaving sufficient to tuck in at the back of the nail.
8. Using the applicator brush, stipple the repair with cement and carefully smooth with solvent using the thumb.
9. Allow the cement to dry before applying the base coat and enamel.

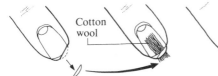

		Trim the tissue
Broken off nail tip apply nail cement to edge of nail tip	Place cotton wool saturated with liquid cement down centre of the nail. Place broken-off nail tip over cotton wool	Turn hand over and trim cotton wool back under the nail	Turn hand over again Bring the cotton wool up from the cuticle and smooth away Place torn tissue saturated with cement over the repair. Trim and tuck tissue under the nail using an orange stick

Fig. 22.4 To re-attach a broken nail

Questions

1. Explain why mending tissue should be torn rather than cut when carrying out a repair.
2. Give three reasons why nails may split or break. What action may be taken to alleviate the problem?
3. Name the materials used in carrying out nail repairs.
4. Explain why the thumb is moistened with nail enamel solvent before smoothing repair patches.
5. At what stage of a manicure are nail repairs carried out?

Chapter 23

Artificial nails

Artificial nails have become increasingly popular over the past few years and are worn to enhance the shape of the nails and the appearance of the fingers and hands. They are available as ready-prepared 'stick-on' type nails, and as 'build-on' or sculptured nails. Artificial nails are bought as a pack or kit and the manufacturer's instructions regarding application must be carefully followed. They may be used to conceal broken nails, improve very short or mis-shapen nails, overcome nail biting and to protect the natural nails from splitting and breaking.

'Stick-on' false nails

These are pre-formed sets of nails in varying shapes and sizes, so that most people should be able to find suitable false nails without having to resort to the excessive shaping and filing which used to be the case. The false nails are made of plastic resins, and a suitable adhesive with which to attach them to the natural nails is supplied with the kit. It is recommended that the nails are worn only for short periods not exceeding 48 hours, in order to keep the natural nails in good condition. They are detachable and may be re-used. Thus false nails are often worn for special occasions or as a fashion accessory. It is even possible to have gold-plated nails or nails set with precious stones.

False nails should never be applied if the surrounding skin or cuticles are infected, inflamed or damaged, or if the natural nail plates show any sign of infection. Before commencing the application, the false nails should be checked for correct size, both in length and width. The client's nails should be grease-free, and the cuticles moulded back to facilitate a better fit of the false nails.

Method of application

1. Remove any old nail enamel from the client's nails and carry out the usual manicure procedure up to but not including the base coat application.
2. Select the appropriate false nails and, using fine emery paper, scratch and roughen them on the underside to facilitate their adhesion.

3. Carry out any trimming or filing required at the cuticle end of the false nails to make them correspond to the shape of the client's own nails.
4. Immerse the false nails in warm water for a few minutes in order to soften them and make them more pliable, so that they can be adjusted to fit the curvature of the client's nails.
5. Dry the nails and place them on a strip of adhesive tape with the concave side uppermost. (Adhesive strip is usually supplied with the nail kit.) Then apply a small amount of adhesive to the edges of the client's nails, and also a fine coat to the concave side of the false nails (see Fig. 23.1). Allow this to dry for about two minutes.
6. Starting with the thumb, press the false nail on to the client's own nail with the base touching or resting just under the cuticle. Apply slight pressure for one minute to effect adhesion. Using an orange stick protected with cotton wool moistened with nail enamel remover,

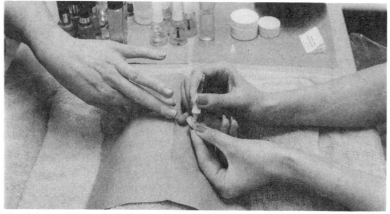

Fig. 23.1 Application of adhesive on a false nail

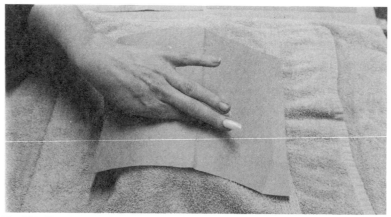

Fig. 23.2 Completed application of false nail

carefully wipe away any excess adhesive. The completed application of a nail is shown in Fig. 23.2.

7. Repeat the procedure until all the nails have been fitted. Allow them to dry thoroughly for about five minutes before applying the base coat and enamel if required.

Note: The adhesive is highly flammable and so should never come into contact with a naked flame. The vapour from the adhesive is toxic and should not be inhaled. The application should take place in a well-ventilated room.

Removal of 'stick-on' nails

'Stick-on' nails are readily detachable and may then be stored for re-use later. After softening the adhesive with a little oily acetone-free enamel remover applied round the edges of the nail, they may be removed by lifting gently with a protected orange stick. Undue force should not be used and, if necessary, enamel remover should be re-applied until the nail can be removed with ease. All adhesive should be cleaned from both the natural and false nails using more enamel remover. The false nails should then be washed and stored on the adhesive strip provided with the kit.

Removal of enamel from false nails

Some plastic resin nails may be dissolved by acetone, therefore any enamel remover used on this type of nail must be acetone-free.

Advice to clients

It may be suggested to the client that she returns to the salon for the removal of false nails. If, however, she intends to remove them herself, the procedure for removal and re-use should be explained. Advice should also be given regarding the care of the nails while being worn.

1. Contact of the nails with any naked flame, e.g. matches, cigarette lighters, and with lighted cigarettes must be avoided.
2. Frequent immersion of the nails in hot water may loosen the nails.
3. Care should be taken not to apply pressure to the tips of the nails as they may be loosened by leverage.
4. The nails should not be worn for more than 48 hours at any one time.
5. The nails should be removed immediately if any signs of allergy, such as inflammation or itching, occur.
6. Nail enamel removers containing acetone should be avoided.

'Build-on' nails (sculptured nails)

This type of artificial nail is formed on the natural nail plate itself during a chemical reaction called *polymerisation*, in which molecules of a substance known as a *monomer* are linked together chemically to form larger molecules of a substance called a *polymer*. The most frequently used monomer is methyl methacrylate, and the sculptured nails thus consist of the corresponding polymer called polymethyl methacrylate (an acrylic resin).

The kit for sculptured nails contains the following:

1. A nail-shaped protective shield which is placed under the natural nail while the nail builder is being used.
2. An application brush.
3. A bottle containing the liquid monomer, methyl methacrylate.
4. A jar of powdered ingredients, including a catalyst (usually benzoyl peroxide), to increase the speed of the reaction, a small quantity of polymer which is necessary to start the reaction, and sometimes a small amount of pigment.

The powdered ingredients are mixed with the liquid monomer immediately before use. The chemical reaction takes place on the natural nail itself, forming a hard film of polymer.

Method of application

'Build-on' nails are applied after a normal manicure has been carried out up to, but not including, the application of the base coat.

1. Place the protective shield underneath the natural nail plate and ensure that it fits firmly and securely (see Fig. 23.3).

(a) Nail before the shield is in place

(b) The metal shield is placed under the free edge of the natural nail

Fig. 23.3 Preparation for 'build-on' nails

2. Mix the powdered and liquid ingredients together to obtain a smooth fluid paste according to the manufacturer's instructions.
3. Starting at the base of the nail and using the brush provided, apply the paste evenly and smoothly along the nail and on to the protective shield in the same way as the application of nail enamel. The manicurist will decide how far to take the application over the nail shield according to the length of nail required (see Fig. 23.4).

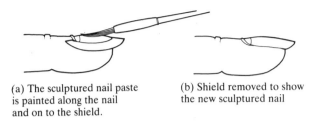

(a) The sculptured nail paste
is painted along the nail
and on to the shield.

(b) Shield removed to show
the new sculptured nail

Fig. 23.4 Sculptured nails completed ready for filing

4. If all the nails are to be treated, carry out the same procedure on each in turn.
5. Allow 10–15 minutes for the chemical reaction to be completed and for the nails to harden before removing the protective shield.
6. File the new nails to the shape required to complement the shape of the client's fingers and hands. A metal file must be used since emery boards are not strong enough for shaping this type of nail.
7. Wash the nails thoroughly and allow them to dry, before applying a base coat followed by nail enamel and top coat.

These nails are a semi-permanent fixture, and new growth of the nails leaves a gap at the base which needs in-filling approximately every two or three weeks. The nails cannot be removed by the client; the manicurist must use an electric nail-drill for their removal.

Contra-indications to the use of 'build-on' nails

1. Inflammation of the tissues surrounding the nails.
2. Cuts and abrasions in surrounding tissue.
3. Diseases or disorders of the nail plate.
4. Allergy to the chemicals used. Methyl methacrylate is a known sensitiser. Allergy may result in inflammation and swelling of the surrounding tissues, and in severe cases the nail may become detached from the nail bed. It is difficult to treat since the artificial nail is not easily removed and takes several months to grow out.

Nail extension

This is a form of artificial nail but does not cover the whole of the nail plate. As the name implies, the free edge of the nail is extended by the false nail to give extra length to the client's nails. Nail extenders are available in kit form which includes a suitable adhesive.

Method of application

1. Ensure that the client's nails are clean and free from grease.
2. Select the appropriate extensions by matching them up with the shape of the client's own nails.
3. Carry out any necessary shaping of the client's nails, in order to obtain a good fit with the nail extension.
4. Using the coarse side of an emery board, roughen the edges of the false nail to encourage greater adhesion.
5. Apply a small amount of adhesive under the overlap at the base of the extension.
6. Position the nail extension on the edge of the client's nail and press firmly until adhesion takes place.
7. Now shape the nail tip and carry out filing and buffing on the nail plate until the surface is smooth.
8. Re-apply the adhesive at the join of the nail extension both on top and underneath the nail. Allow the adhesive to harden and then apply enamel in the usual way.

Note: Always work well away from naked flames. Do not inhale the fumes of the adhesive. Keep the adhesive away from the eyes.

Questions

1. Give three reasons why false nails are worn.
2. For how long would you suggest that false nails of the 'stick-on' variety should be worn? Give reasons for your answer.
3. How may extra length be added to make a client's nails longer?
4. Which type of false nails are considered to be semi-permanent?
5. How would you prepare 'stick-on' type false nails to ensure a good fit?

Chemicals used in manicure

Acetone	Solvent in nail enamels and nail enamel removers (now rarely used).
Acrylic resin	Film former in nail enamels. Used in sculptured nails and nail hardeners.
Amyl acetate	Solvent in nail enamels.
Beeswax	Wax base of nail white pencils.
Bentonite	A clay (hydrous aluminium silicate) added to enamels, especially pearlised enamels, to prevent the separation of ingredients on standing.
Benzoyl peroxide	A catalyst used to speed polymerisation of methyl methacrylate in sculptured nails.
Bismuth oxychloride	Made synthetically or obtained from fish scales. Consists of highly reflective platelets used in pearlised (crystalline) nail enamels.
Butyl acetate	Solvent in nail enamels and nail enamel remover.
Calamine	Pink powder of zinc carbonate. Mixed with rose water and used as a soothing paste for skin irritations on the hands.
Carnauba wax	Hard wax obtained from the surface of palm leaves. Wax base for polishing sticks for buffing. Added to base coat to fill out irregularities in the nail plate.
Castor oil	Ingredient of nail white pencils. Added to nail enamel removers to counteract drying effect of solvents.
Cetyl alcohol	Waxy non-greasy white solid used as an emollient in hand creams.
Ethyl acetate	Solvent in nail enamels and nail enamel remover.
Formaldehyde resin	Film former in nail enamels. Used in nail hardeners. Potential sensitiser.
Fuller's earth	Mixed with rose water for treatment of badly soiled hands.
Glycerol	Humectant and emollient used in cuticle remover and hand creams.

Gum tragacanth	Suspending agent in liquid buffing polishes. Thickener for cuticle remover.
Iron oxide	Inorganic pigment used in nail enamels.
Isopropyl myristate	Plasticiser in nail enamel to make it more flexible on the nail.
Kaolin (China clay)	White slightly abrasive powder used in buffing powders and pastes.
Lanolin	Obtained from sheep's wool. Similar to sebum. Emollient in hand cream, cuticle massage cream, nail enamel removers and nail white pencil. Potential sensitiser.
Magnesium carbonate	Slightly astringent white powder mixed to paste with water for remedial treatment of badly soiled hands.
Methyl cellulose	Suspending agent in liquid buffing polishes. Thickener for cuticle remover.
Methyl methacrylate	Acrylic resin monomer. Ingredient of nail cement for repair work. Also in build-on sculptured nails.
Mineral oil	A petroleum product used in oil phase of hand creams, cuticle massage creams and nail bleach creams. Added to nail enamel removers and nail enamel dryers.
Nitrocellulose	Film former in nail enamel.
Olive oil	Vegetable oil used in oil manicures for ridged and brittle nails. Mixed with bran in cleansing treatments for dry hands.
Paraffin wax	A petroleum product used in remedial treatments for stiff joints.
Petroleum jelly	A petroleum product used in nail bleach creams.
Polymethyl methacrylate	Polymer formed on the nails in build-on sculptured nails.
Potassium hydroxide	Caustic alkali used as cuticle remover.
Pumice	Grey abrasive powder used for buffing very ridged nails. Also as rough stone used to remove stains from the skin.
Rose water	Perfumed water mixed with calamine in treatments for skin irritations.
Sodium hydroxide	Caustic alkali used as cuticle remover.
Stannic oxide	Slightly abrasive powder used for buffing.
Stearic acid	White waxy solid used in hand creams.
Talc	Magnesium silicate. Slightly abrasive powder used for buffing.
Titanium dioxide	Intensely white powder used in nail whitener pastes and pencils, also in nail bleaches.

	Added to cream nail enamels to produce pastel shades.
Toluene	Solvent in nail enamels.
Triethanolamine	Used as cuticle remover as alternative to potassium and sodium hydroxides.
Trisodium phosphate	Used as cuticle remover as alternative to potassium and sodium hydroxides.
Zinc peroxide	Used in nail bleach creams and pastes.

Multiple choice questions for manicure

In each of the following questions, choose the most suitable answer from the four alternatives given.

1. A nail grows from
   (a) the lunula
   (b) epidermal tissue
   (c) dermal tissue
   (d) the nail cuticle

2. The hyponychium lies
   (a) behind the cuticle
   (b) under the lunula
   (c) under the free edge of the nail
   (d) in the nail grooves

3. The function of the cuticle is to
   (a) hide the nail matrix
   (b) grow over the lunula
   (c) protect the skin around the nail
   (d) prevent infection entering the nail fold

4. The cuticle is an extension of
   (a) the stratum corneum
   (b) the stratum lucidum
   (c) the stratum granulosum
   (d) the stratum germinativum

5. Beau's lines on the nail plates are caused by
   (a) serious illness
   (b) fungal infection
   (c) picking at the nails
   (d) hereditary factors

6. The term 'koilonychia' refers to
   (a) brittle nails
   (b) spoon-shaped nails
   (c) ridged nails
   (d) ingrowing nails

7. The term 'paronychia' refers to
   (a) inflammation of the skin surrounding the nail
   (b) allergic reaction to nail enamel
   (c) separation of the nail from the nail bed
   (d) infection of the nail plate by a fungus

8. Which one of the following substances is most likely to cause an allergic reaction?
   (a) acetone
   (b) formaldehyde resin
   (c) carnauba wax
   (d) castor oil

9. Onycholysis may be caused by
   (a) neglect of hang nails
   (b) overgrowth of the cuticle
   (c) infestation by itch mites
   (d) pressure on the free edge

10. If a client suffers from onychophagy this would indicate that
    (a) her nails were discoloured
    (b) she bites her nails
    (c) white spots were present on the nail plate
    (d) the client had a wart on her finger

11. Crystalline enamel contains
    (a) sodium hydroxide
    (b) potassium hydroxide
    (c) bismuth oxychloride
    (d) hydrogen peroxide

12. Cuticle remover may contain
    (a) hydrogen peroxide
    (b) amyl acetate
    (c) acetone
    (d) sodium hydroxide

13. Nail enamel solvent (thinners) may contain
    (a) mineral oil
    (b) ethyl acetate
    (c) formaldehyde resin
    (d) nitrocellulose

14. Stannic oxide is used in
    (a) crystalline enamels
    (b) nail whiteners
    (c) buffing paste polish
    (d) nail strengtheners

15. When shaping the nails, the emery board should be used
    (a) with a sawing action across the whole nail
    (b) from sides to centre in one direction only
    (c) for bevelling the nails only
    (d) across the surface of the nail plate

16. The buffing technique involves
    (a) vigorous strokes from side to side across the nail
    (b) banging the buffer directly on to the nail plate
    (c) buffing in one direction only from base to free edge
    (d) sliding the buffer vigorously around the nail

17. A cuticle knife should be used
    (a) on the free edge only
    (b) on wet nails
    (c) on dry nails
    (d) to push back the cuticles

18. 'Squeaking' should be carried out
    (a) prior to a hand massage
    (b) prior to the application of enamel
    (c) on completion of the manicure
    (d) after carrying out a repair

19. A top coat is used to
    (a) tone down a bright enamel
    (b) protect the cuticle
    (c) give sheen to cream enamels
    (d) give sheen to crystalline enamels

20. Which of the following conditions is contra-indicative to manicure?
    (a) ringworm of the nail
    (b) allergy to nail enamel
    (c) brittle nails
    (d) onychophagy

21. A base coat is used
    (a) on completion of a manicure
    (b) prior to the application of enamel
    (c) only when applying a cream enamel
    (d) only when applying a crystalline enamel

22. The number of bones in the wrist and hand together is
    (a) 8
    (b) 19
    (c) 27
    (d) 29

23. The joints between the bones of a finger are
    (a) gliding joints
    (b) fixed joints
    (c) ball and socket joints
    (d) hinge joints

24. The arteries in the fingers are called
    (a) digital arteries
    (b) radial arteries
    (c) palmar arches
    (d) phalanges

25. Which one of the following massage movements would not be carried out by a manicurist?
    (a) tapotement
    (b) effleurage
    (c) petrissage
    (d) vibro-massage

26. Oil manicure involves the use of
    (a) mineral oil
    (b) silicone oil
    (c) essential oil
    (d) vegetable oil

27. Paraffin wax treatment is beneficial in cases of
    (a) stiffness of the finger joints
    (b) brittle nails
    (c) psoriasis
    (d) dermatitis

28. A nail repair should be smoothed by use of
    (a) cuticle remover
    (b) nail adhesive
    (c) nail enamel
    (d) nail enamel solvent

29. The chemical reaction taking place during the formation of build-on artificial nails is called
    (a) oxidation
    (b) reduction
    (c) polymerisation
    (d) neutralisation

30. Which one of the following is not a type of false nail?
    (a) a sculptured nail
    (b) a bevelled nail
    (c) a nail extension
    (d) a 'stick-on' nail

Answers to multiple choice questions in manicure

Question:	1	2	3	4	5	6	7	8	9	10
Answer:	(b)	(c)	(d)	(a)	(a)	(b)	(a)	(b)	(d)	(b)

Question:	11	12	13	14	15	16	17	18	19	20
Answer:	(c)	(d)	(b)	(c)	(b)	(c)	(b)	(b)	(c)	(a)

Question:	21	22	23	24	25	26	27	28	29	30
Answer:	(b)	(c)	(d)	(a)	(d)	(d)	(a)	(d)	(c)	(b)

Index